THE UGA

ATHLETE'S TRAINING GUIDE

Champions Train to Be Champions

TYSON JOHNSON

INSTAGRAM

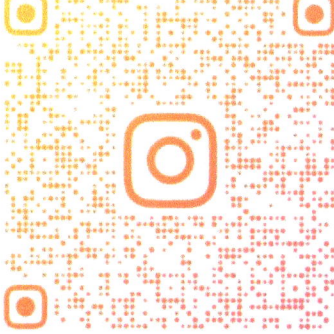

@UNIVERSAL_GRAPPLING_ACADEMY

© 2025 - All Rights Reserved

The UGA Athlete's Training Guide
Mixed Martial Arts, Fitness, Nutrition, and Sports Conditioning

Tyson Johnson
Email: uga@tysonjohnson.com
www.UniversalGrapplingAcademy.com

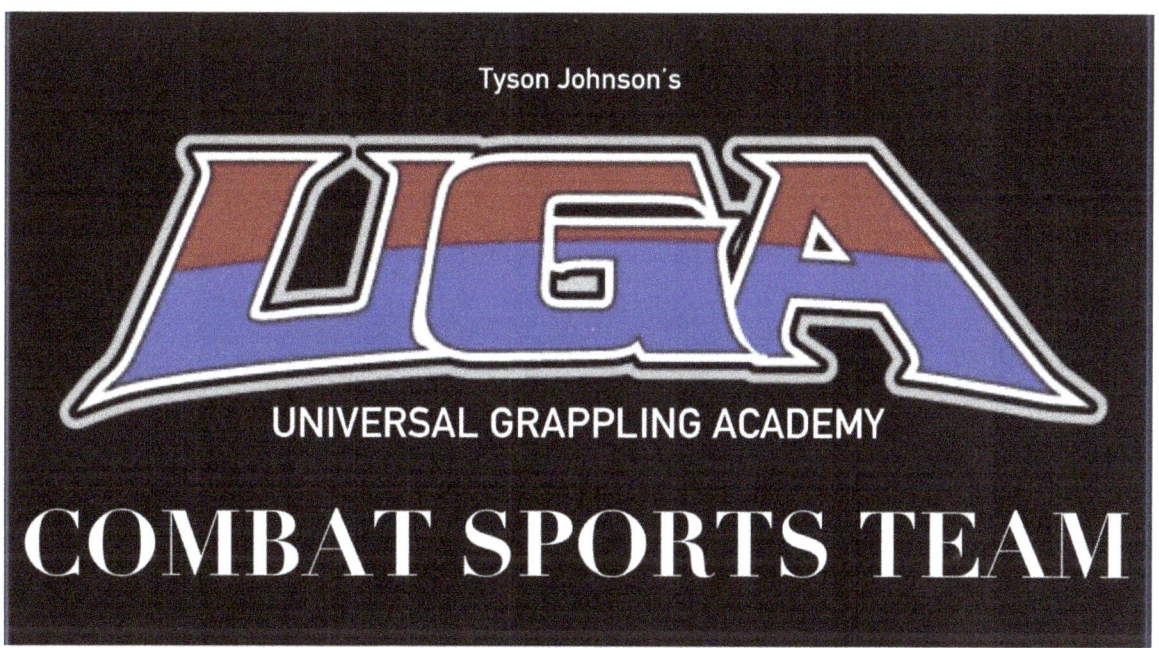

Enjoy your MMA Training:_____
Train Hard & Finish Strong.

Authorized By Coach:_____

"The IronMan" Tyson Johnson

LEGAL NOTICE

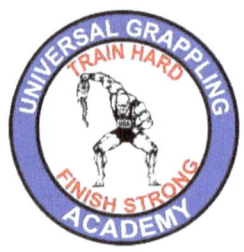

Release of Liability and Disclaimer

Title: The UGA Athlete's Training Guide

Author: Tyson Johnson

Disclaimer:

The information contained in "The UGA Athlete's Training Guide" is intended for educational and informational purposes only. The author, Tyson Johnson, and all publishers or authorized retail agents (collectively referred to as "the Authors") make no representations or warranties of any kind, express or implied, about the completeness, accuracy, reliability, suitability, or availability with respect to the book or the information, products, services, or related graphics contained in the book.

The content contained in this book may not be reproduced, duplicated, or transmitted in any way without the express written permission of the author and - or publisher. You can not amend, distribute, sell, use as your own, quote or paraphrase as your own any part or content contained in this book without the express written consent of the author and or the publisher.

Release of Liability:

By reading this book, you acknowledge and agree to the following:

1. **No Professional Advice:** The content of this book does not constitute professional advice and should not be relied upon as such. The information provided is not a substitute for professional training, guidance, or consultation with a qualified coach, trainer, or healthcare professional.

2. **Assumption of Risk:** Participation in any training, exercise, or athletic activities involves inherent risks, including but not limited to injury or death. You voluntarily assume all risks associated with your participation in any activities described in this book.

3. **Release of Claims:** You hereby release, waive, discharge, and covenant not to sue the Authors for any liability, claims, demands, or causes of action that may arise from your use of the information in this book or your participation in any activities described herein.

4. **Limitation of Liability:** To the fullest extent permitted by law, the Authors shall not be liable for any indirect, incidental, special, consequential, or punitive damages, including but not limited to, loss of profits, data, or use, arising out of or in connection with your use of this book.

5. **Acceptance of Terms:** By reading "The UGA Athlete's Training Guide," you acknowledge that you have read this release of liability and disclaimer, understand it, and agree to be bound by its terms.

This release of liability and disclaimer is effective as of the date of your reading of the book and shall remain in effect for all future reference.

Conclusion: Your participation is entirely voluntary, and you acknowledge that you are solely responsible for your actions and decisions or those of your children.. Always consult with a professional before undertaking any new training, nutrition or exercise program. Thank you for your understanding and for choosing "The UGA Athlete's Training Guide."

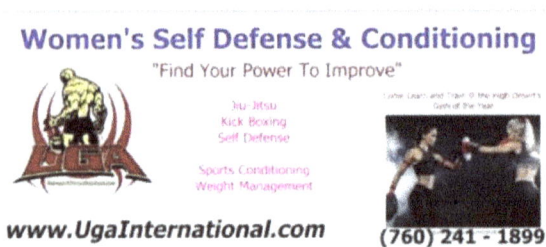

DEDICATION

To all the remarkable men, women, and children who have stepped onto the mats at Tyson Johnson's Universal Grappling Academy over the past three decades, this book is dedicated to you. Your unwavering commitment to growth, resilience, and the pursuit of excellence has transformed not only your lives but also the lives of those around you. Through every sweat-soaked training session, every hard-fought match, and every moment of camaraderie, you have embodied the spirit of dedication and perseverance. May your journeys inspire others to embrace the challenges of life with the same tenacity and passion you have shown. Thank you for being a part of this incredible journey.

It has been my pleasure to "Train Ordinary People to be Extraordinary Athletes."

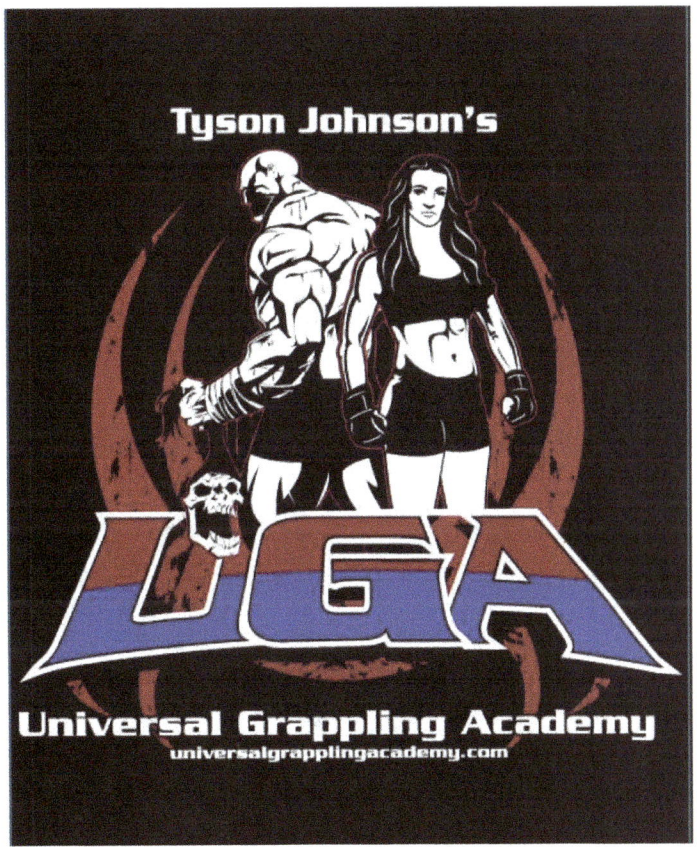

PROLOGUE

In the heart of the High Desert, where the sun casts its warm glow over the rugged landscape, lies a sanctuary for warriors, dreamers, and champions—Tyson Johnson's Universal Grappling Academy. For over thirty years, this facility has stood as a beacon of excellence in combat sports training, a place where passion meets discipline and the pursuit of greatness knows no bounds.

Under the expert guidance of Coach Tyson Johnson, a visionary leader and a master of his craft, the UGA has transformed countless Ordinary People into Extraordinary Athletes. Tyson's dedication to the art of grappling and combat sports is matched only by his commitment to nurturing the spirit of each student. His coaching philosophy goes beyond the physical; he instills values of respect, resilience, and camaraderie, molding not just champions but well-rounded individuals ready to face the challenges of life.

At Universal Grappling Academy, the air is thick with determination and the echoes of hard work. Here, champions are forged through sweat and perseverance, each one a testament to the transformative power of training. From the moment you step onto the mat, you become part of a legacy that celebrates both individual achievement and collective growth. Athletes from all walks of life have walked through these doors, each with their own story, each striving to push the limits of what is possible.

As you delve into the pages of this book, you will discover the training practices of those who have improved at this unparalleled facility, the challenges they faced, and the victories they achieved. You will witness the evolution of ordinary people who became fighters and have risen to greatness, propelled by the unwavering support of coach Tyson and the bond of their training partners. Welcome to the world of the Universal Grappling Academy, where champions are made, and dreams become reality.

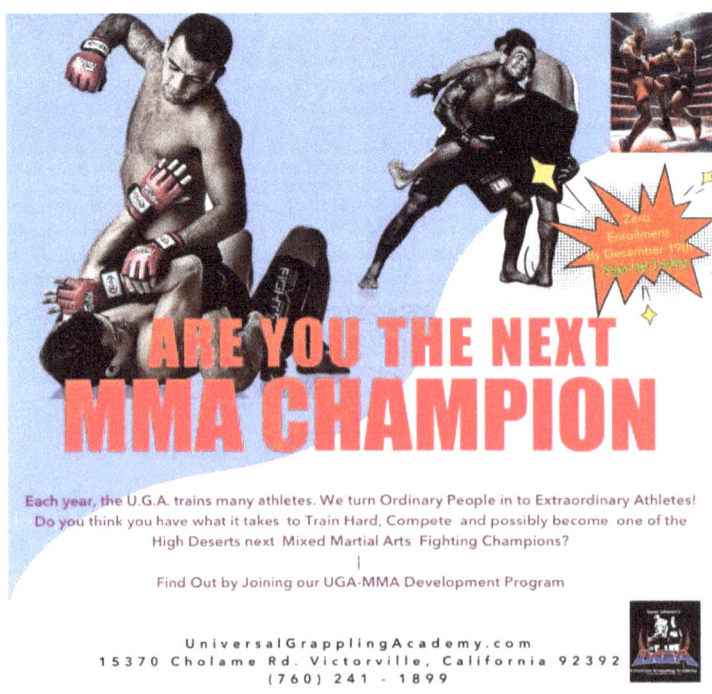

Table of contents

DEDICATION iii
PROLOGUE iv
Chapter 1 1
   Become A UGA Athlete 1
CHAPTER 2 11
   increase Your Fighter IQ 11
CHAPTER 3 14
   Nutrition For Combat Sports 14
CHAPTER 4 25
   mental Toughness & Psychology 25
CHAPTER 5 32
   Humble warriors 32
CHAPTER 6 35
   Extreme self-defense 35
CHAPTER 7 40
   combat Sports Competition 40
CHAPTER 8 58
   Safety And Awareness 58
CHAPTER 9 67
   A Family That Trains Together 67
Chapter 10 72
   Whiteboard Knowledge 72
CHAPTER 11 77
   the Coaches Office 77
CHAPTER 12 83
   UGA Training Routines 83

This Guide Belongs To

Name:_____

Age:_____ Height:_____ Weight:_____

Weight Goal:_____

My Personal Goals: Pick All That Apply

1. **Improved Fitness And Nutrition**
2. **Self Defense / Confidence**
3. **Improved Sports Conditioning**
4. **Improved Combat Sports Knowledge**
5. **Combat Sports Competition**

I understand that i am responsible for my own improvements. By reading, understanding and applying the training and knowledge content in the UGA athletes's training guide, it would be extremely hard for me to fail. I promise myself that i will not procrastinate, be lazy or make excuses to fail. I will do the best that i can to improve myself physically, mentally and emotionally for myself and those in my life.

Personal Promise Acceptance: Yes_____ No_____

CHAPTER 1

BECOME A UGA ATHLETE

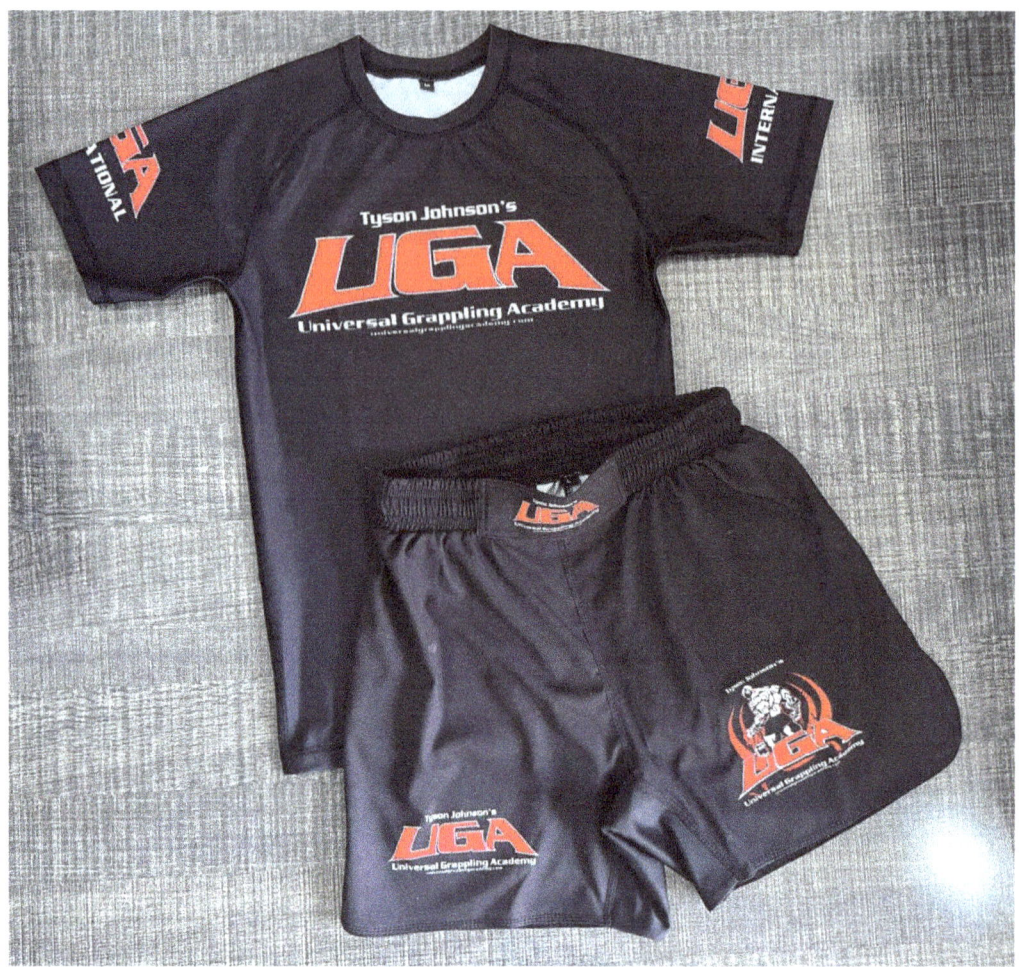

"Training Ordinary People to Be Extraordinary Athletes"

Becoming a UGA athlete involves several steps, focusing on physical training, mental conditioning, and lifestyle choices. Here's a basic guide to help you get started.

 Yes, many will tell you that my training methods are old-school, with rough training systems that put your body through extreme conditions (little rest, breaks and babying), but it works. That's why we've made so many champions, However, as this world gets softer with all these millennial types, things get watered down because they can't handle my old style of IronMan championship training. Do your best and become the best that you can be!

1. Choose Your Sport: Identify that UGA MMA is what you are interested in and really want to do. Consider your strengths, interests, and the level of commitment you are willing to make.

2. Set Goals: Establish short-term and long-term goals. These could range from general fitness, self defense, improving your skills or competing at a certain level.

3. Start Training: Find coach Tyson and join the Universal Grappling Academy training program. Coach Tyson will provide you with structured training, guidance, and feedback on your performance.

4. Develop a Training Routine: Create a consistent training schedule that includes skill practice, strength training, conditioning, and flexibility exercises. Be consistent, don't make excuses and miss practice.

5. Focus on Nutrition: Eat a balanced diet that supports your training needs. This includes proper hydration, and consuming the right amounts of carbohydrates, proteins, and fats.

6. Mental Preparation: Develop mental toughness and focus. Techniques such as visualization, meditation, and positive self-talk can enhance performance. A weak mind will weaken the body. Training won't be easy, if it was was, everyone could do it and you wouldn't be special.

7. Stay Committed: Consistency is key. Stick to your training regimen, even when motivation wanes. Your goals don't care about your excuses. The more you focus and train, the better you'll get.

8. Participate in Competitions: Start competing in class sparring, at grappling tournaments, exhibitions and local mma events to gain experience and assess your progress.

9. Rest and Recover: Allow your body time to recover to prevent injuries. Incorporate rest days and listen to your body. Remember, Being lazy isn't resting and recovering, it's steps backwards from your goals.

10. Seek Feedback: Regularly evaluate your performance and seek feedback from coach Tyson and veteran UGA members to identify areas for improvement.

Remember: as coach tyson always says, *'The Best Way to get through it is to get to it".* becoming a uga athlete is a journey that requires the 3 d's (Desire, dedication, and determination) along with patience and resilience. Enjoy and follow the process so you can celebrate your progress!

Teamwork plays a significant role in Uga-mma training. even though the focus may seem to be on individual performance. Here are several ways in which teamwork impacts individual combat training:

1. Support System: Athletes often rely on coaches, trainers, and teammates for emotional and psychological support. This support can be crucial during training and competitions, helping athletes stay motivated and focused.

2. Training Partners: Many individual sports, such as in MMA, benefit from having training partners. These partners can provide competition, help improve skills, and offer constructive feedback.

3. Shared Knowledge: uga Team members can share insights, techniques, and strategies that can enhance individual performance. Learning from each other can lead to faster improvement and new perspectives. I train people to have the ability to train people.

4. Accountability: Being part of a team can create a sense of accountability. Athletes may push themselves harder in training and maintain discipline when they know others are counting on them.

5. Camaraderie and Motivation: The camaraderie that develops among team members can foster a positive environment. The motivation to succeed alongside peers can drive individuals to strive for excellence. Iron sharpens iron!

6. Specialized Roles: In the Uga, athletes may work with specialized roles within a team, such as sparring partners or strategists, which can enhance their performance.

7. Mental Resilience: Team environments can help athletes develop mental resilience by providing a network of encouragement and shared experiences, which can be beneficial during tough training times.

8. Resource Sharing: The UGA team can pool resources, such as access to our training facilities, equipment, and additional coaching, which can enhance the overall development of individual athletes.

UGA teamwork in mma contributes to an athlete's overall development, performance, and enjoyment, emphasizing that even solo combat sports activities often thrive with the support and collaboration of others.

Building A Strong Mind to be a Champion

Building a championship mindset at the Universal Grappling Academy with Coach Tyson Johnson begins with cultivating discipline, resilience, and a relentless pursuit of excellence.

Start by setting clear, achievable goals that challenge your limits while remaining realistic; this will provide motivation and a sense of direction. Embrace a growth mindset by viewing setbacks as opportunities for learning and improvement, fostering a positive attitude even in the face of adversity.

Regularly engage in intense training sessions, pushing yourself physically and mentally while also being open to feedback from Coach Tyson, who emphasizes the importance of technique and strategy.

Surround yourself with a supportive community of fellow grapplers who uplift and inspire you, fostering a collaborative environment that enhances your training experience.

Ultimately, consistency in practice, mental fortitude, and a commitment to your personal development will help you embody the championship mindset essential for success in the Universal Grappling Academy.

"Everything Starts with a Strong Mind. If you have a strong mental attitude and mindset, your body will follow. Think Strong, and you'll train strong so you can become strong."

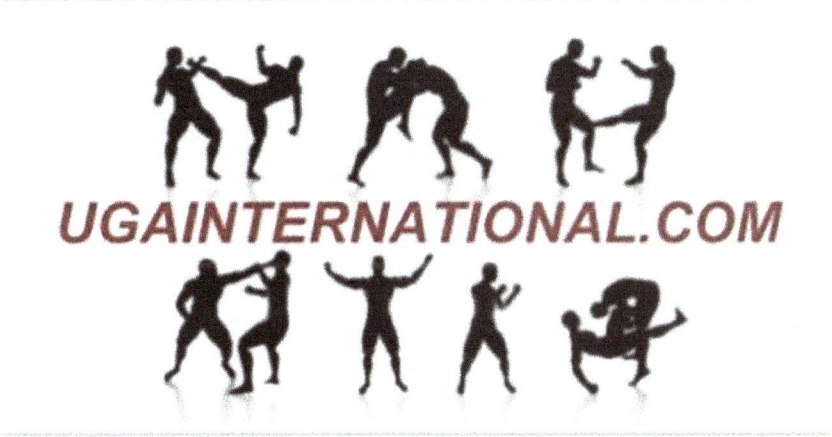

Champions train to be champions

Training to become a champion in grappling, mixed martial arts (MMA), or combat sports requires a well-rounded approach that encompasses physical conditioning, technical skills, mental fortitude, and strategic planning. Here are some key components to consider:

The 3 D's

1. *Desire* - To achieve and be successful in everything you do as a UGA student. Nothing comes easy; if you really want something, you'll work for it.

2. *Dedication* - Be dedicated to your goals. You must commit to yourself and your future. If you're not dedicated to your goals, how can you expect youR coaches to be?

3. *Determination* - be determined to reach your goals through consistent training and constant learning of your craft. If you want it, you'll get it as long as you stay determined to get it. Let nothing stop you.

1. Skill Development: Focus on mastering the fundamental techniques of grappling and striking. Regularly practice various submissions, escapes, takedowns, and striking techniques, ensuring you have a strong foundation in both disciplines.

2. Physical Conditioning: Prioritize strength, endurance, flexibility, and agility through a tailored UGA fitness program. Incorporate cardiovascular training, weightlifting, and mobility exercises to enhance your overall physical performance.

3. Sparring and Live Drilling: Engage in regular sparring sessions to apply techniques in real-time scenarios. This helps develop timing, distance management, and the ability to adapt to an opponent's movements.

4. Mental Resilience: Cultivate a champion's mindset by practicing visualization, positive self-talk, and stress management techniques. Develop the ability to stay calm under pressure and learn to embrace adversity as part of the journey.

5. Nutrition and Recovery: Maintain a balanced diet that supports your training regimen and promotes recovery. Prioritize hydration, proper nutrition, and adequate sleep to optimize performance and prevent injury.

6. Coaching and Feedback: Work closely with experienced UGA coaches who can provide guidance and feedback. Regularly assess your performance and be open to constructive criticism to continually improve.

7. Strategy and Game Planning: Analyze opponents and develop fight strategies tailored to your strengths and weaknesses. Being tactical in your approach can give you a significant advantage in competition.

8. Consistency and Dedication: Commit to a regular training schedule, ensuring that you consistently put in the hard work required to improve. Dedication to your goals, your training routine and yourself is crucial for long-term success.

9. Adaptability: Be prepared to adjust your techniques and strategies based on your opponents and the evolving nature of the sport. Flexibility in your training approach is essential to stay competitive.

10. Community and Support: Surround yourself with supportive UGA team members. Having training partners and mentors who share your goals can motivate you and provide valuable insights.

By integrating these keys into your training regimen, you can lay the groundwork for becoming a successful grappling or MMA champion. Consistency, dedication, and a commitment to continuous improvement are vital to achieving your goals in the Universal Grappling Academy and combat sports.

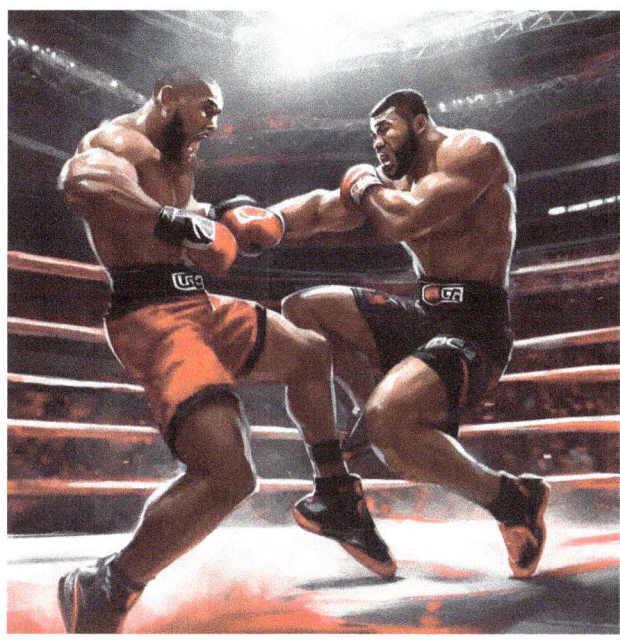

You may be unaware, but just by reading this first chapter, you've already begun your journey of uga training. I say this because, if you haven't noticed, I've laid out some of our basic principles a couple of times in the same or slightly different way. Part of your UGA training is about finding your personal learning patterns.

Not everybody learns at the same pace or in the same way, but the best way to get something to be a natural movement and part of your muscle memory is to go over it and practice it many times over....I'm talking about "repetition"; the more you do something, the sooner it can become a part of who you are and as a natural part of your movements. The same goes with your reading patterns; if i say it multiple times, the sooner it'll stick in your brain and will become who you are as a future UGA athlete and champion.

The thing is, People learn differently; while some are visual learners, others are Physical learners, some are slow learners, while others pick things up immediately. Some students need to go over a move many times, while others will get it after seeing it just once.

This being the case, a good coach needs to be able to adapt and change their training methods to the various types of learning abilities of their students. Find out what type of teaching works best for the different types of student and their individual abilities.

You have four months to Learn, Practice, and Have a good Understanding of Positions, Offensive & Defensive moves.

Things to Remember: As a UGA Level 8 Athlete

3 –D 's

1. Desire – To Learn & Improve my Health, Fitness, and Emotional Status.
2. Determination – To Continue Working Hard & Take Steps Towards my Goals.
3. Dedication – To Attend Class, Focus, and Apply my Moves to the Best of my Ability.

EXERCISES: Jumping Jacks / Sprawls / Push-Ups / Cube Jumps / Front Rolls / Frog Leaps / Shrimp Drills / Squats / Lunges / Guard Defense / Spin Drill / Neck Bridge / Hip Up-Out-Bump /Duck Walks

POSITIONS: Full Mount / 5-Star Post / Side Mount (elevated & flat) / Knee Post / Back Mount / Seat-Belt Back Control / North-South / Open Guard / Closed Guard / Butterfly Guard / Half Guard / Z-Guard /

STANCES: Staggered Stance / Square Stance / Low Stances

TIE-UPS: Close Collar / Extended / Bear Hug / Double-Over / Over-Under / Clinch

TAKE-DOWNS: Single Leg / Double Leg / Ankle Pick / Knee Pick / Head & Arm /

SUBMISSIONS: Basic – CP Arm Bar / Axe Choke / Guillotine Choke / Rear Naked Choke / Key Locks / Kimura/

TRANSITIONS: Take-Down to Control Position / Tie-Up Duck-Under to Seat Belt /

ESCAPES: Guard / Full Mount / Side Mount / Seat Belt /

From all basic positions, we can expand the moves, transitions, and submissions as the students advance.

Things to Remember: As a UGA Level 7 Athlete

3 Points of Balance – Control these points standing or on the ground, and you'll have better control over your opponent's balance.

1. Head – Leads the direction of the body / Where the head goes, the body goes.
2. Shoulders – Directs the upper body flow, angle, and balance.
3. Hips – The base core which controls the flow and balance of the lower body.

EXERCISES: Duck Walk / Basic 4 point Foot Movement and Pivoting / Clinch / Knee / Push Kick / Jab / 1-2 Punch / Bob & Weave / Block / Cover-Up / Lean Back / Elbows /

POSITIONS: Full Mount / 5-Star Post / Side Mount / Knee Post / Back Mount / Seat-Belt Back Control / North-South / Open Guard / Closed Guard / Butterfly Guard / Half Guard / Z-Guard /

STANCES: Staggered Striking / Horse Stance / Plank

TIE-UPS: Pummel / Close Collar / Extended / Bear Hug / Double-Over / Over-Under / Clinch / Half Clinch /

TAKE-DOWNS: Hip Toss / Monkey Roll / Belly to Belly Dump / Belly to Back Dump / Leg Trip

SUBMISSIONS: Wrist Lock / Top Position – Face Plant (Mounted) Arm-Bar / Side-Mount(Knee-Post) Arm-Bar / Side-Mount Step-Over Arm-Bar / Inverted Arm-Bar (locks) from Side-Mount / Bottom Position – Arm-Bar from Guard / Arm Lock / Triangle-Choke /

TRANSITIONS: Take Down to Control Position to Arm-Bar to a Wrest Lock / Triangle Choke to an Arm-Bar to a Wrist Lock /

ESCAPES: Sit-Out / Standing- Ground Switch / Head & Arm Lock

UNIVERSAL GRAPPLING ACADEMY
Rank Divisions

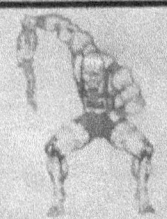

DIVISION#   **Techniques, Moves, and Applications**

8 - Beginner Stances-wrestling, kickboxing, **Tie ups**-wrestling, double over, double under, over under, **Mount** full mount, side mount, sidemount escape, 5 star defense, **Guard**-full guard, half guard, passing the guard, **Chokes**-Axe guillotine, rear naked, **Key Locks**-side mount 3 arm position, kimura, **ArmBar**-c.p. armbar

---

7 – White **Takedowns**-single, double, head & arm, hip toss, monkey roll, pummel leg trips, sprawls (body-push-away), **ArmBars**-face plant, reverse (inverted), arm locks, sidemount armbar, tri-angle choke, triangle to armbar, **Leg-Locks**-figure four, heal hook, knee bar, knee lock, head and arm takedown, 5min Match.

---

6 – Yellow Referee's position, sit-out, switch, standing grip break, standing kimura, sit through kimura, ostritch roll, chin lock, stepover from guard, gator roll, sidemount leg lock, double axe choke, grape popper from guard (bicep strangle), wrist lock, leg locks from opponent standing guard or butterfly guard 5min Match

---

5 – Orange **Wall takedowns**-double, single, outside leg hook, inside leg hook, mounted armbar from choke distraction, knee bar from half guard, hip toss, north/south armbar, oma plata, jab, double jab, one/two, clinch, knee, thrust kicks, kick check, elbow strikes, uppercut, strike defense, 5min Match

---

4 – Blue Answer fundamental list questions, demonstrate random moves, disrupt opponent attack, demonstrate pain points, sidemount arm locks, must pass against 1 opponent **Hunter Program** – leg lock, armbar, choke 2 – 5min Matches

---

3 – Purple combinations of takedowns, trap, control, positions, submissions, show ability to improvise against various opponent attacks, 2 opponent hunter program, striking combinations, chin choke, 10 minute ironman match vs division 2 opponent,

---

2 – Brown striking combinations and techniques, 3 opponent hunter program, disrupt opponent attack vs division 2 opponent, 10 minute ironman match, demonstration of various moves, run 3 classes – techniques, striking, and conditioning

---

1 – Black demonstration of all moves (offense & defense), written explanation of UGA fundamentals, transitions of moves and combinations, explain the application of various moves, 4 opponent hunter program, ground and pound demonstration, run 3 classes – technique, striking, and conditioning, 15min Ironman match

---

To Qualify – 132 Actual Training Days in the Universal Grappling Academy Training Center & Show Understanding of Techniques as well as be able to effectively apply both Offensive and Defensive Moves. Upper levels must also be able to demonstrate transitions and combinations of moves. Regular and Ironman matches should be against an opponent of another training facility. Winning Tournament matches qualify.

CHAPTER 2

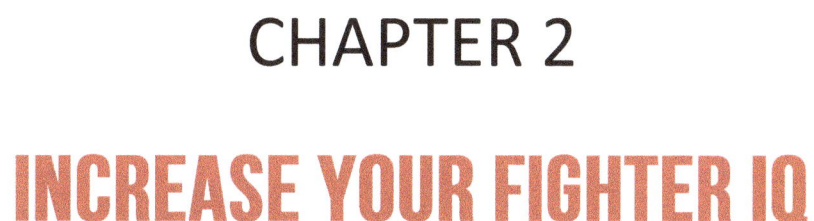

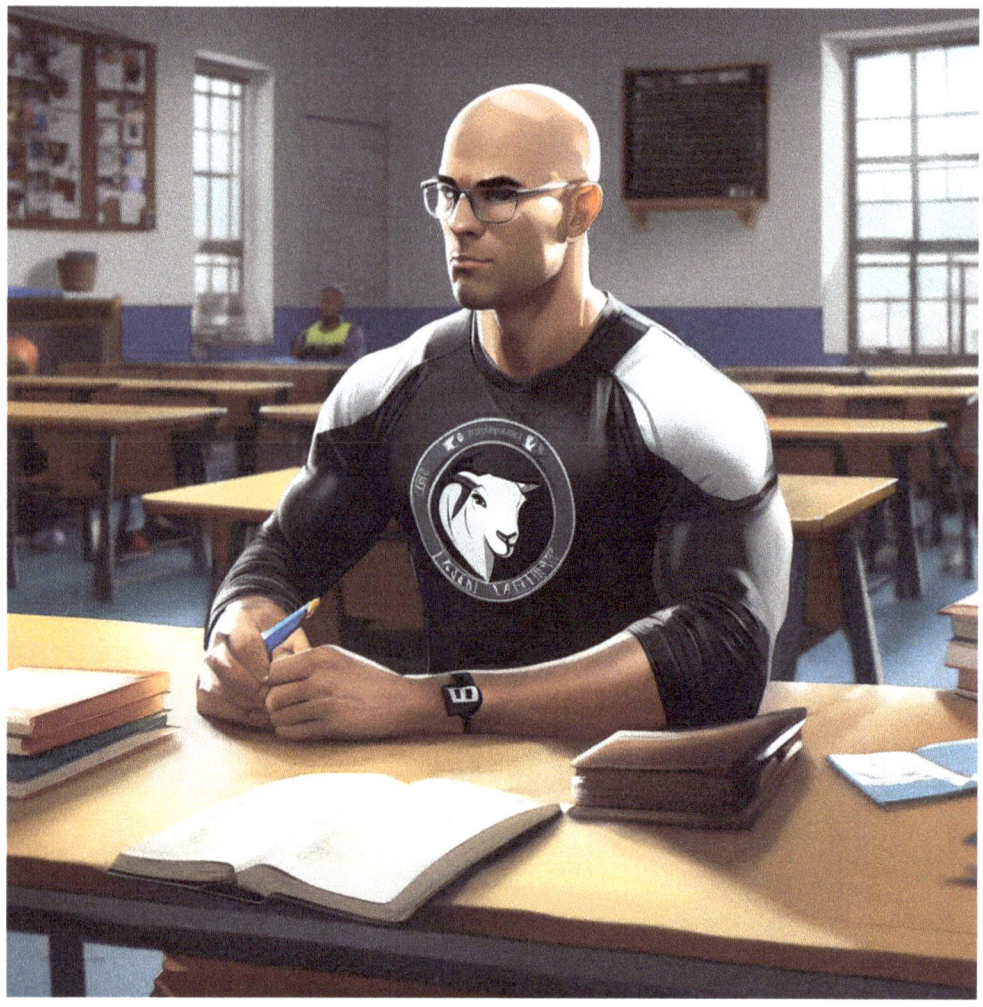

Knowledge is Power; the more that you know, the more powerful you'll be in your combat sports journey. Improving your combat sports IQ / knowledge involves a combination of education, observation, and practice.

1. Study Techniques and Fundamentals: Dive into the basic techniques of various combat sports (MMA, Boxing, Wrestling, Jiujitsu, Judo, etc.) through training at the UGA, instructional videos, books, and online courses.

Understanding the fundamentals is crucial and can help develop a better understanding of who you are or will be as a combat sports athlete.

2. Watch Fights: Analyze professional matches. Pay attention to strategies, footwork, defense, and how fighters adapt to their opponents. Taking notes can help reinforce what you observe.

3. Follow Experts: Engage with content created by experienced fighters, coaches, and analysts. Podcasts, YouTube channels, and social media platforms often feature breakdowns of techniques and fight strategies.

4. Train Regularly: Practical experience is invaluable. Join the Universal Grappling Academy training facility, where you can practice techniques, spar with others, and receive feedback from coaches.

5. Join Discussion Forums: Participate in online communities or forums dedicated to combat sports. Engaging in discussions can provide new insights and help you learn from others' experiences. Take in as much information and different views, but pick and choose what works best for you.

6. Attend Live Events: Watching live events such as the Gladiator Challenge, LightsOut Xtreme Fighting, the UFC, One Fighting Championships, Bare Knuckle Fighting etc. This can provide a different perspective and enhance your understanding of the sport. Pay attention to the atmosphere, techniques, and how fighters interact with their environments.

7. Study Sports Psychology: Understanding the mental aspects of combat sports, such as mindset, strategy, and confidence, can significantly improve your approach to training and competition.

8. Cross-Training: Explore other martial arts or combat sports. This can provide a broader perspective on techniques and strategies that might be applicable to your main discipline. The great thing about training at the UGA is that we train in MMA (mixed martial arts), which trains you in a wide variety of combat arts to assist you in this process, from various stand up and ground techniques.

9. Keep a Journal: for some students, by documenting your training sessions, insights from fights, and strategies you learn. Reflecting on your notes can solidify your understanding and track your progress.

10. Seek Feedback: Regularly ask for feedback from coaches and peers on your techniques and strategies. Constructive criticism can help you identify areas for improvement.

By combining these methods, you can significantly enhance your combat sports IQ and overall performance.

CHAPTER 3

NUTRITION FOR COMBAT SPORTS

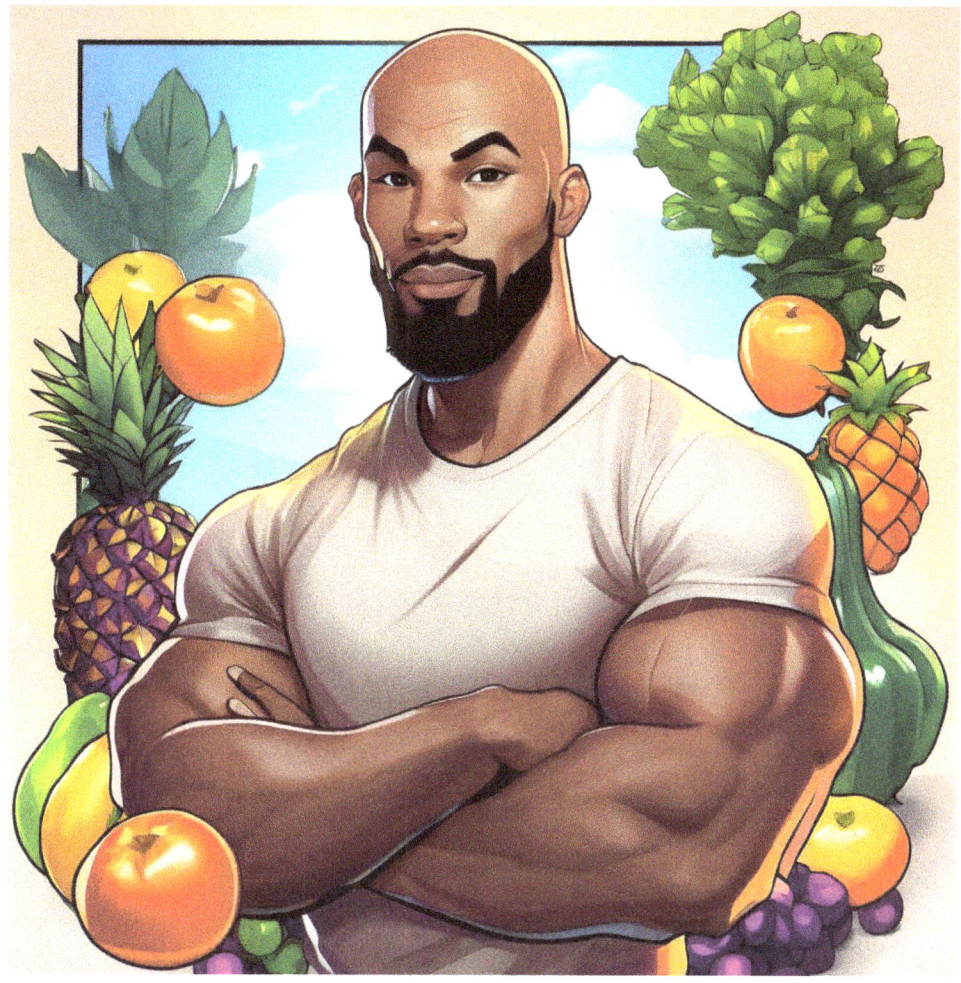

Nutrition plays a crucial role in a combat athlete's performance in combat sports for several reasons:

1. Energy Levels: Proper nutrition provides the necessary energy for training and competition. Athletes require a balanced intake of carbohydrates, fats, and proteins to fuel their workouts and maintain stamina throughout fights.

2. Muscle Recovery: Adequate protein intake is essential for muscle repair and recovery after intense training sessions. Consuming protein-rich foods helps to rebuild muscle fibers and reduce soreness.

3. Hydration: Staying hydrated is vital for optimal performance. Dehydration can lead to fatigue, decreased focus, and impaired physical performance. Athletes must drink enough fluids (water, coconut water) before, during, and after training and competition.

4. Weight Management: Many combat sports have weight classes, so managing body weight is crucial. Athletes need to follow specific nutrition strategies to lose or maintain weight while ensuring they still have the energy to perform at their best.

5. Immune Function: Intense training can weaken the immune system. A well-balanced diet rich in vitamins and minerals supports immune health, helping athletes stay healthy and avoid illness that could disrupt training.

6. Mental Focus: Nutrition also impacts cognitive function. A diet that includes essential nutrients can enhance focus, reaction time, and overall mental clarity, which are vital during competition.

7. Performance Optimization: Specific nutrients can enhance performance. For example, consuming carbohydrates before a fight can provide quick energy, while electrolytes help maintain muscle function and prevent cramps.

8. Long-Term Health: A balanced diet contributes to overall health, reducing the risk of injuries and chronic diseases. This longevity in health is important for an athlete's career and quality of life.

9. Timing of Nutrient Intake: The timing of meals and snacks can affect performance. Consuming the right nutrients at strategic times (e.g., pre-workout, post-workout) can maximize energy levels and recovery.

10. Individualization: Each athlete has unique nutritional needs based on their body type, training intensity, and goals. Tailoring nutrition plans to individual requirements can significantly enhance performance.

In summary, nutrition is a foundational aspect of an athlete's training regimen in combat sports, influencing energy levels, recovery, mental focus, and overall performance. Proper dietary choices can lead to better training outcomes and competitive success.

Here's a deeper look into the role of nutrition for combat sports, emphasizing specific components, strategies, and how they affect performance:

1. Macronutrients:
Carbohydrates: These are the primary energy source for athletes. They are stored as glycogen in muscles and the liver, providing energy during high-intensity workouts and competitions. Complex carbohydrates (like whole grains, fruits, and vegetables) are preferred for sustained energy, while simple carbohydrates (like fruits and sports drinks) can provide quick energy when needed.

Proteins: Essential for muscle repair and growth, proteins also play a role in hormone production and immune function. Athletes should aim for lean protein sources such as chicken, fish, eggs, dairy, legumes, and plant-based proteins. Post-workout protein intake, ideally within 30 minutes, can enhance recovery.

Fats: Healthy fats are a crucial energy source, especially during prolonged, low-intensity exercise. Sources like avocados, nuts, seeds, and olive oil provide essential fatty acids that support overall health and hormone production.

2. Micronutrients:
Vitamins and minerals: play significant roles in energy production, bone health, and muscle function. For example, calcium and vitamin D are vital for bone strength, while B vitamins are crucial for energy metabolism. Antioxidants (such as vitamins C and E) help reduce oxidative stress from intense training.

3. Hydration:
Hydration: is critical for maintaining performance levels, especially in combat sports where weight cutting is common. Dehydration can lead to decreased strength, endurance, and cognitive function. Athletes

should monitor their fluid intake and consider electrolyte balance, especially after intense workouts or competitions.

4. Weight Management:
Many combat sports require athletes to compete within specific weight classes. Effective weight management strategies involve:
- *Caloric Deficit:* Gradually reducing calorie intake to lose weight while preserving muscle mass.

- *Meal Timing:* Planning meals around training sessions to optimize performance while managing weight.

- *Weight Cutting Techniques:* Using safe methods to lose water weight temporarily before weigh-ins, followed by rehydrating properly before competition.

5. Meal Planning:
Pre-Workout Nutrition: Eating a balanced meal with carbohydrates and protein 2-3 hours before training can enhance performance. A small snack, like a banana or a protein bar, can be consumed 30-60 minutes prior for an energy boost.

Post-Workout Recovery: A combination of protein and carbohydrates after training helps replenish glycogen stores and repair muscle tissue. For example, a smoothie with protein powder, fruits, and spinach can be an effective recovery meal.

6. Supplements:
While a well-rounded diet should provide most nutrients, some athletes may consider supplements like protein powders, creatine, or branched-chain amino acids (BCAAs). It's important to consult with a nutritionist or dietitian before adding supplements to ensure they are appropriate and effective.

7. Psychological Effects:
Nutrition: can also impact an athlete's mental state. A well-nourished athlete is more likely to have higher energy levels, better mood, and improved focus. Conversely, poor nutrition can lead to fatigue, irritability, and decreased motivation.

8. Personalization:
Every athlete is unique, and factors such as age, gender, training intensity, and metabolic rate should inform individual nutrition plans. Working with a sports nutritionist can help tailor a diet plan that aligns with specific goals and needs.

9. Cultural and Ethical Considerations:
Some athletes may follow specific diets due to cultural or ethical beliefs (e.g., vegetarianism or veganism). It's essential to ensure that these diets are balanced and provide all necessary nutrients for optimal performance.

10. Long-Term Approach:
Instead of focusing on short-term diets or quick fixes, athletes should adopt a long-term approach to nutrition. Building healthy eating habits and making gradual changes can lead to sustained performance improvements and overall well-being.

Nutrition is an important part of an athlete's training and performance in combat sports. By focusing on a balanced diet, hydration, and individualized strategies, athletes can optimize their physical and mental capabilities, ultimately leading to better performance in the ring or octagon.

Athlete's Eating Program

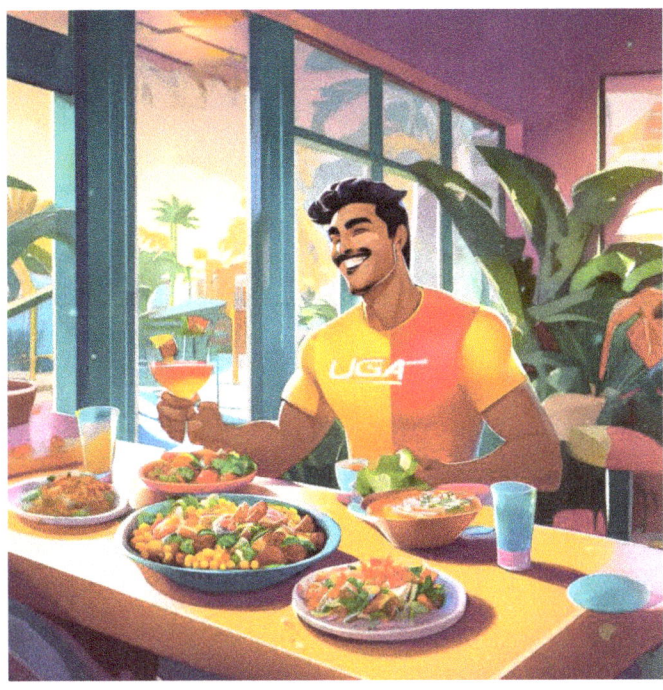

Weight Loss / Fat Burning

Creating an effective eating routine for weight loss and body fat reduction involves focusing on nutrient-dense foods, controlling portion sizes, and maintaining a balanced diet.

General Guidelines
1. **Hydration:** Drink plenty of water throughout the day (aim for at least 8 cups). Herbal teas and black coffee can also be included.
2. **Meal Frequency:** Aim for three main meals and 1-2 healthy snacks per day.
3. **Portion Control:** Be mindful of portion sizes. Use smaller plates if necessary.

Eating Routine

Breakfast (7:00 - 9:00 AM)
- *Option 1:* Greek yogurt with berries and a sprinkle of nuts or seeds.
- *Option 2:* Oatmeal topped with sliced banana and a drizzle of honey or maple syrup.
- *Option 3:* Scrambled eggs with spinach and tomatoes, served with whole-grain toast.

Morning Snack (10:30 - 11:30 AM)
- *Option 1:* A piece of fruit (e.g., apple or pear) with a tablespoon of almond or peanut butter.
- *Option 2:* Carrot or cucumber sticks with hummus.

Lunch (12:30 - 2:00 PM)
- *Option 1:* Grilled chicken or chickpea salad with mixed greens, cherry tomatoes, cucumbers, and a vinaigrette dressing.
- *Option 2:* Quinoa bowl with black beans, corn, diced peppers, avocado, and lime dressing.
- *Option 3:* Turkey or veggie wrap in a whole grain tortilla with lettuce, tomatoes, and mustard.

Afternoon Snack (3:30 - 4:30 PM)
- *Option 1:* A small handful of nuts or seeds.
- *Option 2:* Greek yogurt or a protein shake.

Dinner (6:00 - 8:00 PM)
- *Option 1:* Baked salmon with steamed broccoli and sweet potatoes.
- *Option 2:* Stir-fried tofu or chicken with mixed vegetables and brown rice.
- *Option 3:* Zucchini noodles with marinara sauce and lean ground turkey or lentils.

Evening Snack (optional, if hungry)
- *Option 1:* Air-popped popcorn (lightly salted).
- *Option 2:* A small piece of dark chocolate (70% cocoa or higher).

Additional Tips:
- *Focus on Whole Foods:* Prioritize fruits, vegetables, lean proteins, whole grains, and healthy fats.
- *Limit Processed Foods:* Reduce intake of sugar, refined carbohydrates, and high-calorie snacks.
- *Mindful Eating:* Eat slowly and pay attention to hunger cues; stop when you feel satisfied, not full.
- *Meal Prep:* Consider preparing meals in advance to avoid unhealthy food choices during busy days.

Mass Building Program

Building muscle mass requires a focused eating program that prioritizes high-protein foods, healthy fats, and complex carbohydrates.

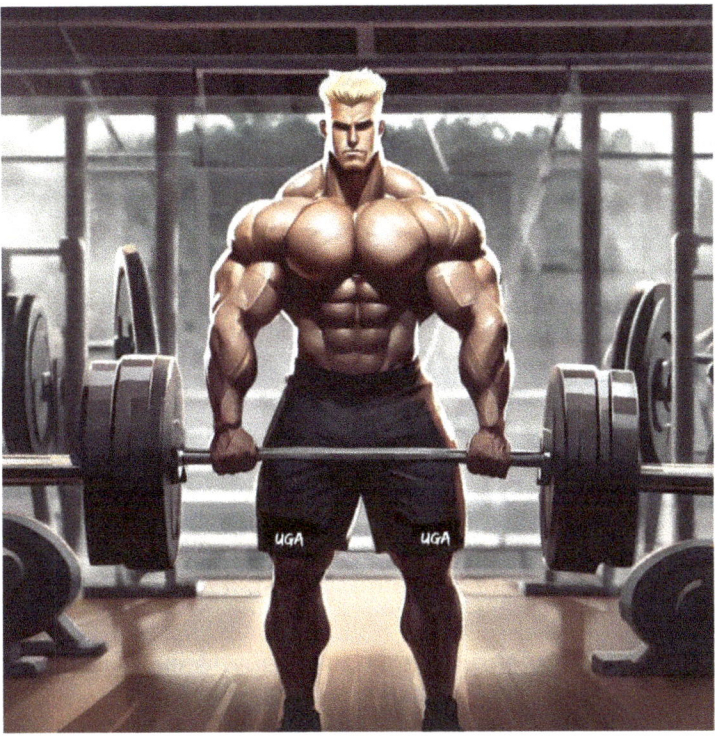

General Guidelines:
1. **Caloric Surplus:** Consume more calories than your body burns to support muscle growth.
2. **Protein Intake:** Aim for at least 1.2 to 2.2 grams of protein per kilogram of body weight.
3. **Meal Frequency:** Eat 4-6 meals per day to ensure a steady intake of nutrients.
4. **Hydration:** Drink plenty of water throughout the day.

Muscle Mass Building Eating Program

Breakfast (7:00 - 8:00 AM)
- *Option 1:* 3 scrambled eggs with spinach and feta cheese, served with whole grain toast and avocado.
- *Option 2:* Oatmeal made with milk, topped with banana, almond butter, and a scoop of protein powder.
- *Option 3:* Smoothie with Greek yogurt, mixed berries, spinach, and a scoop of protein powder.

Morning Snack (10:00 - 11:00 AM)
- *Option 1:* Cottage cheese with pineapple or berries.
- *Option 2:* Protein bar or shake.

Lunch (12:30 - 1:30 PM)
- *Option 1:* Grilled chicken breast with quinoa, mixed vegetables, and olive oil dressing.
- *Option 2:* Turkey or beef stir-fry with brown rice and assorted vegetables.

- *Option 3:* Lentil salad with chickpeas, bell peppers, and feta cheese.

Afternoon Snack (3:00 - 4:00 PM)
- *Option 1:* Hard-boiled eggs with a handful of almonds.
- *Option 2:* Whole grain crackers with hummus or guacamole.

Dinner (6:00 - 7:00 PM)
- *Option 1:* Baked salmon or tilapia with sweet potatoes and steamed broccoli.
- *Option 2:* Grilled steak or chicken thighs with brown rice and sautéed spinach.
- *Option 3:* Pasta with lean ground turkey, marinara sauce, and a side salad.

Evening Snack (8:30 - 9:30 PM)
- *Option 1:* Greek yogurt with a drizzle of honey and mixed nuts.
- *Option 2:* Casein protein shake or cottage cheese with fruit.

Additional Tips:
- *Focus on Whole Foods:* Incorporate lean proteins, whole grains, healthy fats, and plenty of fruits and vegetables.
- *Healthy Fats:* Include sources of healthy fats such as avocados, nuts, seeds, and olive oil to support calorie intake.
- *Post-Workout Nutrition:* Consume a protein-rich meal or shake within 30-60 minutes after workouts to aid recovery.

Meal Prep: Prepare meals in advance to ensure you have ready-to-eat options that align with your goals.

CARDIO-CONDITIONING PROGRAM

An optimal eating program for cardio conditioning should focus on providing the right balance of macronutrients (carbohydrates, proteins, and fats) to support energy levels, recovery, and overall performance.

Daily Meal Structure

1. Breakfast:
  - *Carbohydrates:* Oatmeal or whole grain toast
  - *Protein:* Greek yogurt or eggs
  - *Fats:* A small handful of nuts or avocado
  - *Fruits:* Berries or a banana for quick energy

2. Mid-Morning Snack:
  - *Carbohydrates:* A piece of fruit (like an apple or orange)
  - *Protein:* A small serving of cottage cheese or a protein shake

3. Lunch:
  - *Carbohydrates:* Quinoa or brown rice
  - *Protein:* Grilled chicken, turkey, tofu, or fish
  - *Vegetables:* A large salad with mixed greens, bell peppers, and other colorful veggies
  - *Fats:* Olive oil dressing or a sprinkle of seeds

4. Afternoon Snack:
  - *Carbohydrates:* Whole grain crackers or rice cakes
  - *Protein:* Hummus or nut butter
  - *Vegetables:* Carrot sticks or cucumber slices

5. Dinner:
  - *Carbohydrates:* Sweet potatoes or whole grain pasta
  - *Protein:* Lean beef, fish, or legumes
  - *Vegetables:* Steamed broccoli, spinach, or any seasonal veggies
  - *Fats:* A drizzle of olive oil or a few slices of avocado

6. Evening Snack (optional):
  - *Carbohydrates:* A small bowl of air-popped popcorn or a piece of dark chocolate
  - *Protein:* A scoop of casein protein or a small serving of yogurt

Hydration:
- Drink plenty of water throughout the day. Aim for at least 2-3 liters, depending on your activity level.
- Consider electrolyte drinks during long cardio sessions.

Additional Tips:
- *Timing:* Eat a balanced meal 2-3 hours before cardio workouts for optimal performance.
- *Post-Workout Nutrition:* Consume a mix of carbohydrates and protein (like a banana with a protein shake) within 30-60 minutes after your workout for recovery.
- *Listen to Your Body:* Adjust portion sizes and food choices based on your energy levels and how your body responds to different foods.

Additional Tips:

CHAPTER 4

MENTAL TOUGHNESS & PSYCHOLOGY

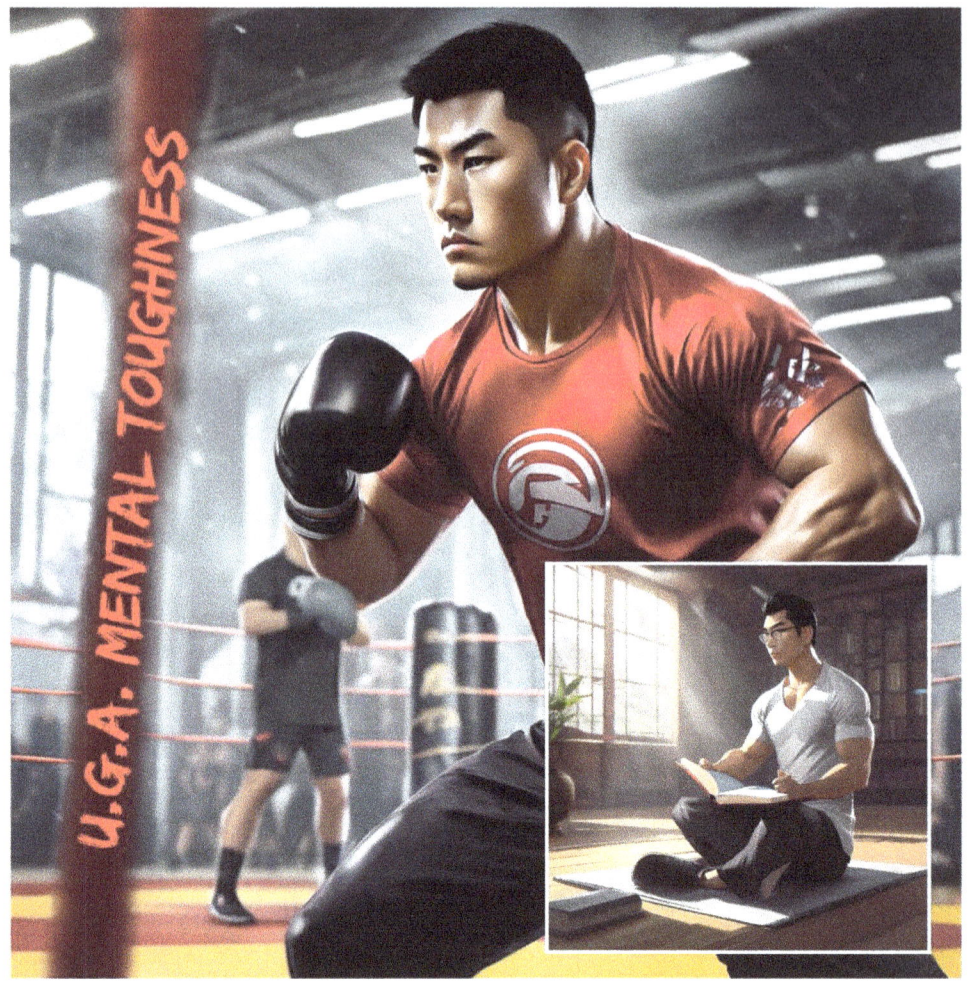

Mental toughness and psychology play crucial roles in the performance of athletes at the Universal Grappling Academy (UGA).

Many people have come in and said that they wanted to compete. But, when it was time to train, or they actually get out there and compete, It's at that point they change their mind and/or start making excuses.

Mental Toughness

1. Resilience: UGA Athletes must develop the ability to bounce back from setbacks, whether it's a loss in a match or a tough training session. This involves maintaining a positive outlook and learning from mistakes.

2. Focus and Concentration: Staying focused during training and competition is essential. Techniques like visualization and meditation can help athletes maintain their concentration under pressure.

3. Confidence: Building self-confidence through consistent practice, setting achievable goals, and celebrating small victories can empower athletes to perform at their best.

4. Discipline and Commitment: Mental toughness requires a strong sense of discipline. UGA Athletes should adhere to training schedules, nutrition plans, and recovery protocols.

5. Stress Management: Learning to cope with stress and anxiety is vital. Techniques such as deep breathing, meditation, or even talking to your coach can help athletes manage their emotions.

Psychological Preparation

1. Goal Setting: UGA Athletes should set short-term and long-term goals. This creates a roadmap for their training and competition, providing motivation and direction.

2. Visualization: Imagining successful performances can enhance confidence and prepare the mind for actual competition. Believe in yourself and your training. UGA Athletes can visualize techniques, outcomes, and their approach to matches.

3. Positive Self-Talk: Encouraging internal dialogue can combat negative thoughts. UGA Athletes should practice affirmations and remind themselves of their capabilities.

4. Routine Development: Establishing pre-competition routines can help athletes enter a focused and calm state. This might include warm-up exercises, breathing techniques, or listening to music.

5. Mental Rehearsal: Practicing scenarios mentally can help athletes prepare for various situations they might face in competitions, enhancing adaptability and response.

Preparation Strategies

1. Consistent Training: Regular practice is fundamental. UGA Athletes should engage in both physical conditioning and technical skills training to enhance their performance.

2. Nutrition and Recovery: A balanced diet and adequate rest are critical for mental and physical performance. Athletes should prioritize nutrition and recovery strategies.

3. Seek Guidance: Working with UGA coaches, sports psychologists, or mentors can provide valuable insights and strategies for mental preparation and performance enhancement.

4. Teammate Support: Building a supportive community among UGA teammates can foster a positive environment where athletes encourage each other and share experiences.

5. Adaptability: Being open to change and willing to adjust training, fighting/grappling styles, and strategies based on performance feedback is essential for growth.

By focusing on these aspects, athletes at the Universal Grappling Academy can enhance their mental toughness and psychological readiness, leading to improved performance and personal growth.

STRESS RELIEF THROUGH TRAINING

The Silent Killer of Motivation, Dedication, and Dreams

As we all know, life can be extremely stressful in so many ways. There is almost nothing more dangerous to destroying your motivation, dedication to your training goals, and/or dreams like daily stress. Of course, not all stress is bad, but in reality, it's all about how you react to the stress in your life that can make the difference. I've had many people thank me for having the UGA in their lives because it was such a stress reducer, and that has always made me happy to hear. Stress can mean and affect people in different ways and evokes a generalized physiological response of the body to physical, psychological, or environmental demands.

I like to use the analogy of "QuickSand"....Stress or other bad situations can and will persist if you sit in it and dwell. However, if you do positive things that will allow you to pull yourself out of the quicksand, then you can create a positive personal atmosphere that'll move you past the negative situation(s). Pick yourself up and pull yourself out!

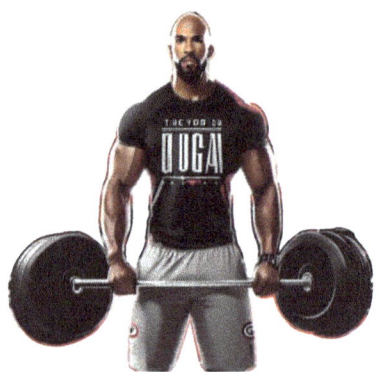

Things that can cause stress in your life and affect your training and/or other daily activities, including happiness.

- Death of a loved one
- Family conflicts
- A serious illness or accident
- Hating your job, position or lack thereof
- Getting fired or laid off from work
- Separation or Divorce proceedings
- Bad fitness or weight management
- A seemingly lack of time or organizational skills
- Bf/Gf Breakup
- Too much responsibility in your life
- Lack of support from family/friends
- Relationships - pre or current marriage
- Loss of personal property

❖ New Job, Driving/Traffic issues, Dealing with People at work or just in life, Having a baby, and so much more…

Stress can manifest in various ways, both physically and emotionally. Here are some warning signs:

1. Emotional Symptoms:
   - Anxiety or constant worry
   - Irritability or mood swings
   - Feeling overwhelmed or helpless
   - Difficulty concentrating or making decisions

2. Physical Symptoms:
   - Headaches or migraines
   - Muscle tension or pain
   - Fatigue or low energy
   - Sleep disturbances, such as insomnia or oversleeping

3. Behavioral Symptoms:
   - Changes in appetite or weight
   - Increased use of alcohol, drugs, or tobacco
   - Social withdrawal or isolation
   - Neglecting responsibilities, training or work

4. Cognitive Symptoms:
   - Memory problems
   - Racing thoughts
   - Difficulty focusing or staying on task

Recognizing these signs early can help in managing stress effectively. If these symptoms persist, it may be beneficial to talk to your coach, spouse, close confidant, or a professional.

Ways to Reduce Stress

As I mentioned before, one of the best ways to reduce stress is to Exercise. Your causes of stress may be mental, but through exercise, you can help reduce it by exercising and physical activities such as UGA-MMA Training. Remember:

Exercising is a good Diversion that enables you to relax and take your mind off your issues by changing your environment and/routine.

MMA Training at the UGA can help dissipate your negative emotions such as frustration, fear, or anger. If you're feeling better mentally due to physical exhaustion, you'll feel better physically. Also if you look better to yourself, it can trigger more positive emotions mentally.

Training produces a biochemical change in your body, which can alter your psychological state of mind. MMA Training may increase the secretion of endorphins in the brain, which helps improve your mood. Normally, people who are fit are in good spirits and feel even better after exercising. This strengthens your ability to fight stress.

Learning to relax and self-talk/meditate is another option to add to your stress relief process. Remind yourself of the good things in your life and figure out a plan to eliminate stress that is bringing you down.

Since stress comes in so many ways, and can be very dangerous to an individual, both mentally and physically, I want to give you a good list of alternate ways to help reduce or eliminate stress.

1. Exercise Regularly: Physical activity can boost endorphins and improve mood. Aim for at least 30 minutes of moderate exercise 3+ days weekly.

2. Practice Mindfulness or Meditation: Techniques like deep breathing, mindfulness meditation, or yoga can help calm your mind and reduce anxiety.

3. Maintain a Healthy Eating Program: Eating a balanced diet rich in fruits, vegetables, whole grains, and lean proteins can improve overall well-being.

4. Be Sure to Get Enough Sleep: Aim for 7-9 hours of quality sleep per night to help your body and mind recover.

5. Establish a Productive Routine: Having a structured daily routine can provide a sense of control and predictability.

6. Have Fun and Stay Connected: Spend time with friends and family, or talk to someone you trust about your feelings.

7. Set Boundaries: Learn to say no and prioritize your time for fun/productive activities that are important to you.

8. Engage in Hobbies: Find activities that bring you joy or relaxation, whether that's UGA training, racquetball, hiking, reading, gardening, painting, or any other hobby. Replace the stress with something positive, convince your mind that you are improving and getting through your issues. Stay positive and you'll be positive.

9. Limit Caffeine and Alcohol: Reducing intake of stimulants and depressants can help stabilize your mood and energy levels.

10. Last Resort - Seek Professional Help: If stress becomes overwhelming, you're having feelings of self-harm or harming others and talking to your coach, family or trusted friend hasn't helped, then consider talking to a therapist or counselor for support and strategies tailored to your needs.

Hopefully, some or all of these practices can help create a more balanced and less stressful life.

Together, we'll Defeat Stress, 1 Rep at a Time. Train Hard/Finish Strong!

CHAPTER 5

HUMBLE WARRIORS

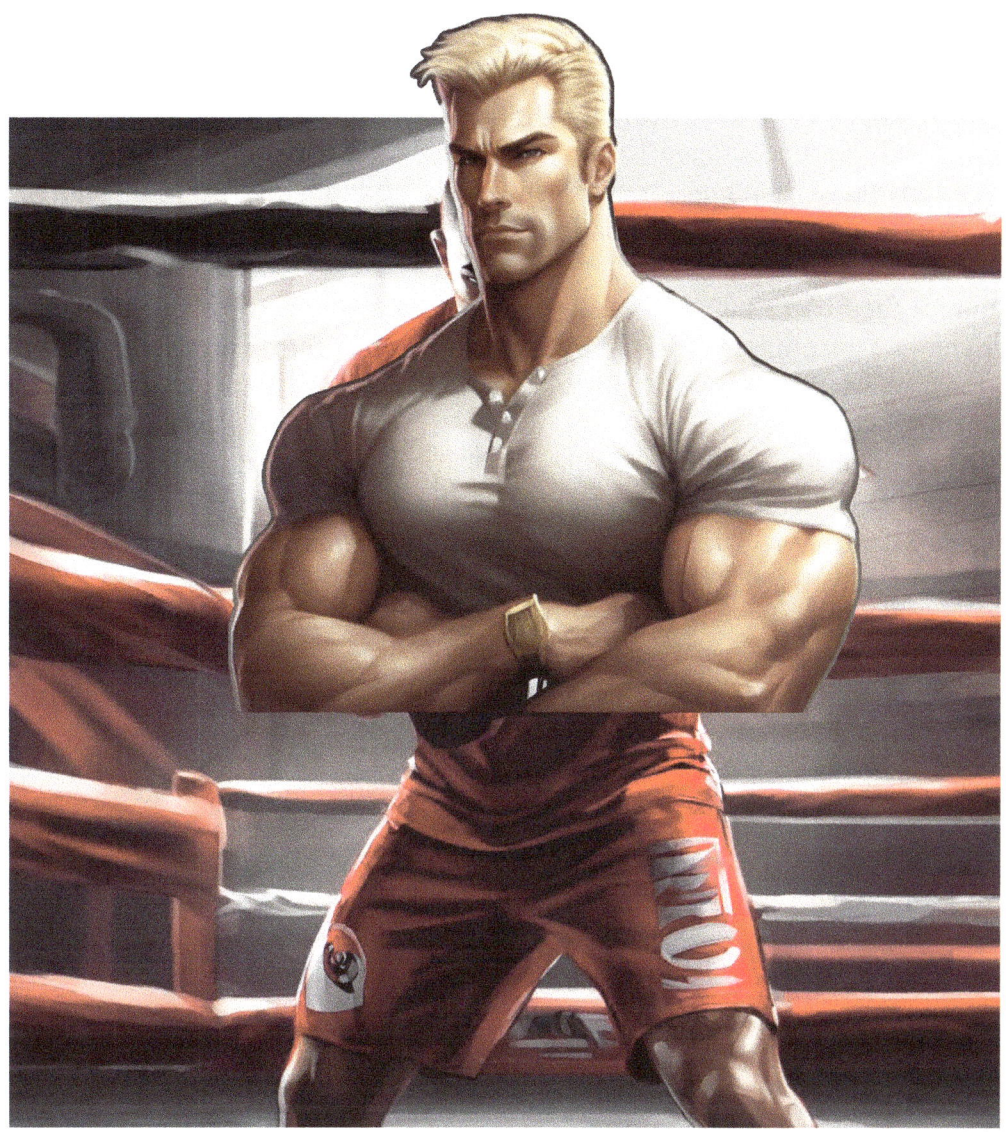

No matter how good you are or are getting, it's always important to stay humble. Confidence is good but cockiness is a buzz kill and a lack of personal strength. Have respect for your opponents, your teammates, your friends and family, the people around you, and of course for your Coach / Training Facility. It's about having self-control, discipline, a good attitude, knowing how to control your anger, and picking your battles. Stay humble and let your actions do the talking for you in and out of competition.

A UGA champion athlete embodies not only physical prowess but also the qualities of humility, self-control, and discipline. Humility is essential because it grounds them, reminding them that their success is often built on the support of coaches, teammates, and their community. By acknowledging these contributions, they set a powerful example for others, showing that their greatness was not achieved all by themselves.

Self-control is crucial in the high-pressure environment of competitive sports. A truly great athlete knows how to manage their emotions, whether in victory or defeat. Maintaining composure, especially during challenging moments, allows them to think clearly and make better decisions, both in their performance and in interactions with others. This self-discipline extends beyond the field; it reflects in their training regimen, lifestyle choices, and commitment to continuous improvement.

A positive attitude is a hallmark of a humble champion. They inspire those around them with their optimism and resilience, even when faced with adversity. This positivity fosters a supportive environment where teammates feel valued and encouraged to push their limits. Furthermore, controlling anger is vital; a champion understands that losing their temper can lead to poor decisions that may affect not only their performance but also their reputation and relationships.

Knowing how to pick their battles is another sign of a true champion. They recognize when to engage in conflicts and when to let go, prioritizing long-term goals over short-term skirmishes. This strategic mindset allows them to focus on what truly matters, further exemplifying their maturity and leadership.

In essence, a UGA champion athlete who embodies humility, self-control, discipline, positivity, and strategic thinking serves as a role model for others. Their ability to rise above challenges while maintaining grace and respect for others is what truly sets them apart, inspiring future generations to not only strive for greatness in their sport but to do so with integrity and humility.

CHAPTER 6
EXTREME SELF-DEFENSE

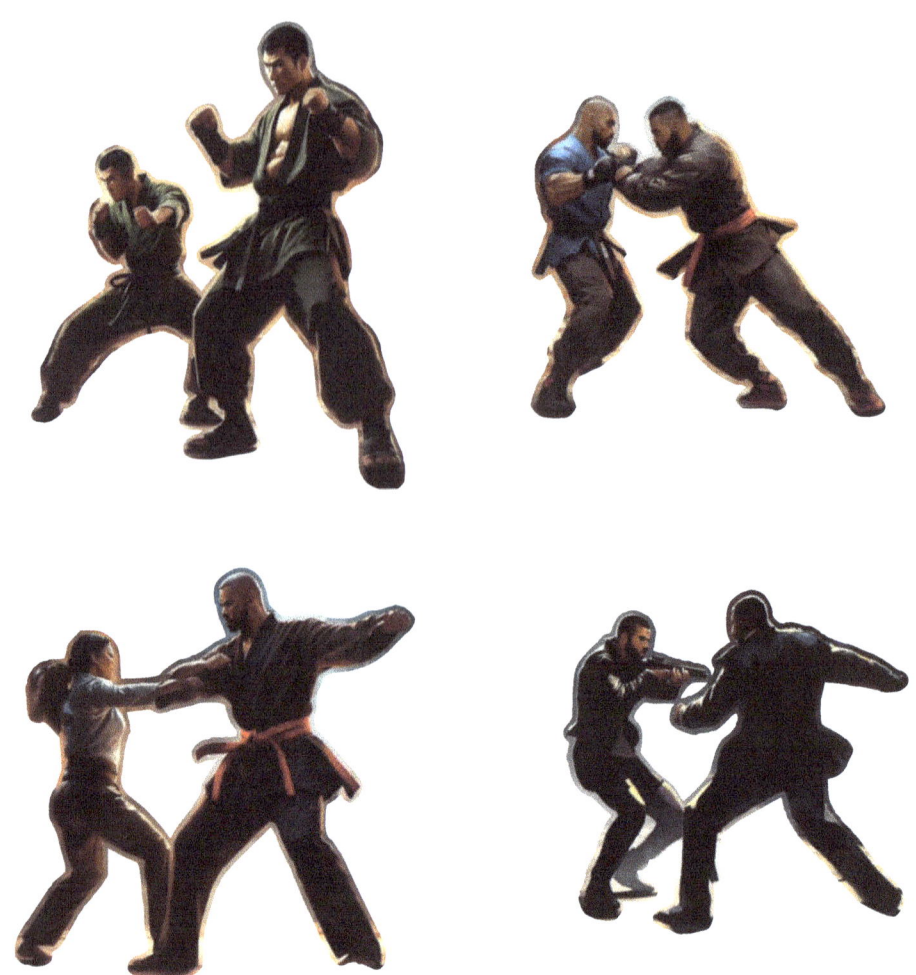

When it's time to protect yourself and or others outside of competition, it's time to "Save a Life" in self-defense. This is where, if necessary, your skills take a temporary dark turn for self-preservation.

If an unfortunate situation and dare I say dangerous situation was to come up, there are still things for you to consider, such as the local laws of self defense actions, using verbal judo to win your battle and if need be, know that a fast and aggressive offensive is best used with "Direct Self-Defense Moves".

As long as you're not the aggressor or bully in the situation, you can effectively and legally defend yourself against an assailant who attacks you. This does not necessarily give you the right to kill; there is a 'Use of Force" law that you should follow, which states that you can and should only use the amount of force necessary to defend/protect yourself against an aggressor. As soon as you can get away, you should do so and seek help.

Utilizing your UGA (Universal Grappling Academy) skills for extreme self-defense outside of competition can be a valuable asset in ensuring personal safety. However, it's crucial to approach this responsibility with a clear understanding of local self-defense laws and the appropriate use of force.

Understanding Local Self-Defense Laws

Before considering any self-defense measures, familiarize yourself with the self-defense laws in your area. These laws vary significantly; some jurisdictions allow for a reasonable level of force in self-defense situations, while others might have stricter regulations. Generally, the use of force must be proportional to the threat faced. For example, if confronted with verbal aggression, responding with physical force is often not justified. Understanding these nuances can protect you legally and ensure that your actions are appropriate for the situation.

Using Verbal Judo

In many aggressive encounters, the initial confrontation can be diffused through effective communication. "Verbal Judo" is a technique that emphasizes using words to de-escalate potentially violent situations. Some strategies include:

1. Empathy: Acknowledge the aggressor's feelings without agreeing with their actions. For instance, saying, "I understand that you're upset," can sometimes help to lower their defenses.

2. Redirecting: Instead of confronting aggression head-on, steer the conversation towards a more constructive dialogue. Phrases like, "Let's take a moment to think this through," can help in shifting the tone.

3. Staying Calm: Your demeanor can influence the aggressor's behavior. Remaining composed and speaking calmly can often reduce tension.

4. Setting Boundaries: Clearly communicate your stance. Use assertive language to set boundaries, such as, "I don't want any trouble. Let's walk away."

If verbal tactics fail and an aggressor becomes physically threatening, it's crucial to be prepared to protect yourself.

Using UGA Skills for Defense

If the situation escalates and the aggressor puts their hands on you, use your UGA skills effectively. Focus on fast, aggressive, and direct moves to neutralize the threat and create an opportunity to escape. Here are some key points to consider:

1. Target Vulnerable Areas: Use strikes to vulnerable points, such as the eyes, throat, or groin, to incapacitate the aggressor momentarily.

2. Quick Movements: Employ swift, decisive techniques that emphasize speed and efficiency. The goal is to create distance between you and the aggressor.

3. Leverage Techniques: Utilize striking and grappling moves to control or off-balance the opponent. Techniques such as footwork, fast/accurate strikes, joint locks, or throws can help to gain the upper hand.

4. Always Prioritize Escape: The primary objective in any self-defense scenario is to escape safely. Once you have neutralized the immediate threat, prioritize getting away from the situation and contacting your parents, teachers, or law enforcement.

By combining an understanding of local laws, effective verbal communication skills, and decisive physical techniques, you can navigate potential threats with confidence. Remember, self-defense is not just about fighting; it's about ensuring your safety while being aware of your legal and moral responsibilities.

Here's a list of extreme self-defense moves that can be effectively used from your UGA training, including kickboxing, boxing, wrestling, judo, jiu-jitsu, Kung Fu San Su, and Krav Maga:

Kickboxing
1. Roundhouse Kick: A powerful kick aimed at the opponent's legs, head, or body, effective for maintaining distance.
2. Teep Kick (Front Kick): A quick push kick that can disrupt an opponent's balance or create space.
3. Knee Strike: A close-range strike targeting the opponent's groin, abdomen, or face, especially effective in clinch situations.

Boxing
1. Jab: A quick, straight punch to keep an opponent at bay and assess their movements.
2. Cross: A powerful straight punch that can be thrown after a jab to create openings.
3. Uppercut: An upward punch aimed at the chin, effective in close range to catch opponents off guard.

Wrestling
1. Double Leg Takedown: A fundamental move that involves taking the opponent down by grabbing both legs.
2. Single Leg Takedown: Similar to the double leg, but focusing on one leg to bring the opponent down.
3. Sprawl: A defensive move used to counter takedown attempts, involving spreading the legs back and lowering the hips.

Judo
1. Ippon Seoi Nage (One-Arm Shoulder Throw): A throw that uses the opponent's momentum to flip them over your shoulder.
2. O Goshi (Hip Throw): A powerful throw that uses your hip to lift and throw the opponent.
3. Kesa Gatame (Scarf Hold): A control position that can be used to immobilize an opponent on the ground.

Jiu-Jitsu
1. Rear Naked Choke: A submission technique applied from behind, effectively incapacitating an opponent.
2. Armbar: A joint lock that hyperextends the arm, used to control or submit an opponent.
3. Triangle Choke: A choke applied using the legs, creating a triangle around the opponent's neck and one arm.

Kung Fu San Su
1. Palm Strike: A powerful strike using the palm to target sensitive areas like the nose or chin.
2. Low Sweep Kick: A kick aimed at the opponent's legs to destabilize them, often used to set up other attacks.
3. Joint Locking Techniques: Various techniques to manipulate an opponent's joints, creating pain or immobilization.

Krav Maga
1. Hammer Fist: A downward striking motion that can target various areas, including the head or collarbone.

2. Defense Against Choke: Techniques to break free from various choking scenarios, often involving strikes and body positioning.

3. Groin Kick: A targeted strike to the groin area, effective for incapacitating an opponent quickly.

These moves can be adapted for self-defense scenarios, focusing on quick, efficient techniques to neutralize threats. Always prioritize safety and practice these techniques responsibly.

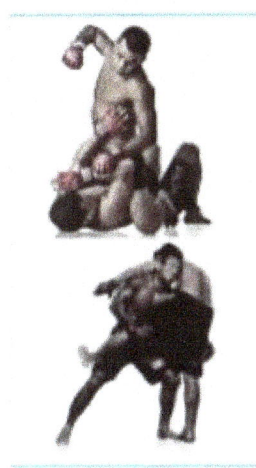

CHAPTER 7

COMBAT SPORTS COMPETITION

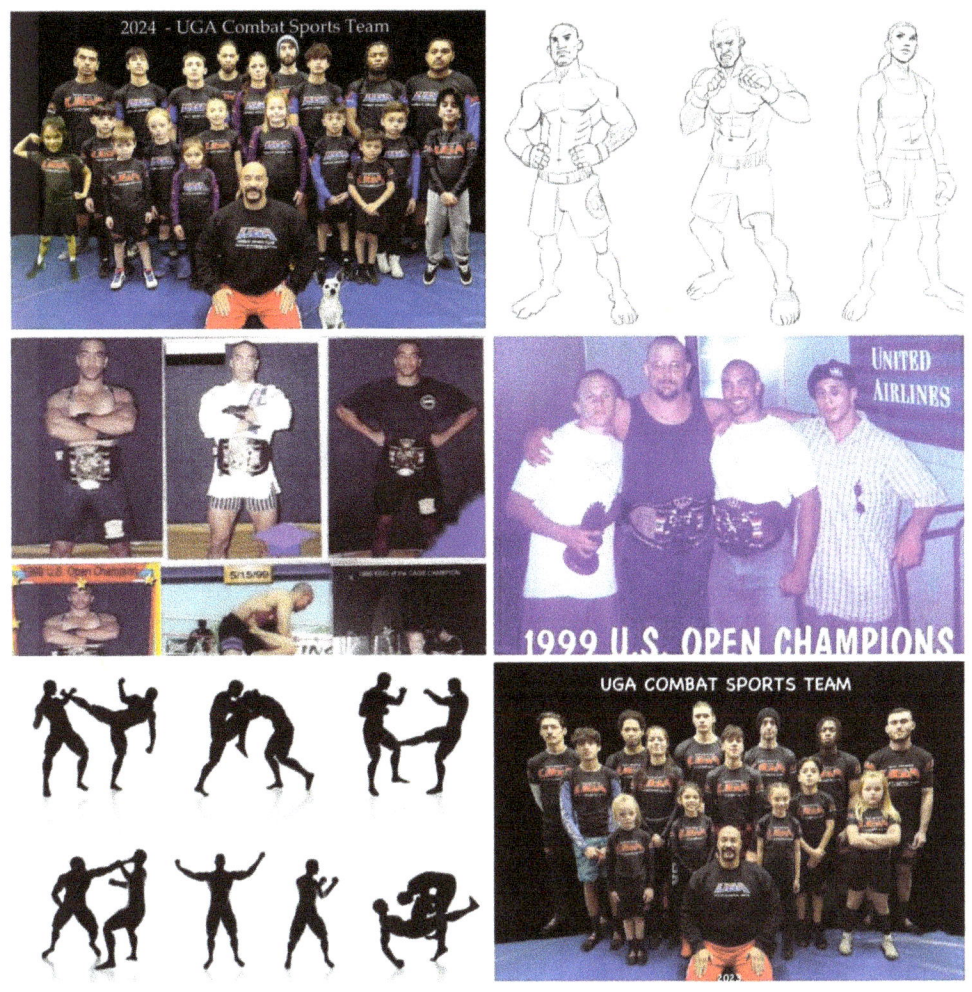

This chapter can provide a comprehensive guide for UGA students interested in joining our Combat Sports Team and the knowledge necessary for optimal performance.

Mixed Martial Arts = A combination of 2 or more arts: Wrestling, Judo, Jiujitsu, Muay Thai, Boxing, Kickboxing, Tae Kwon Do, Karate, Sambo etc.

Sports Combat Competition = the use of one or more of these can be used in schools, the Olympics, tournaments, rings or cages.

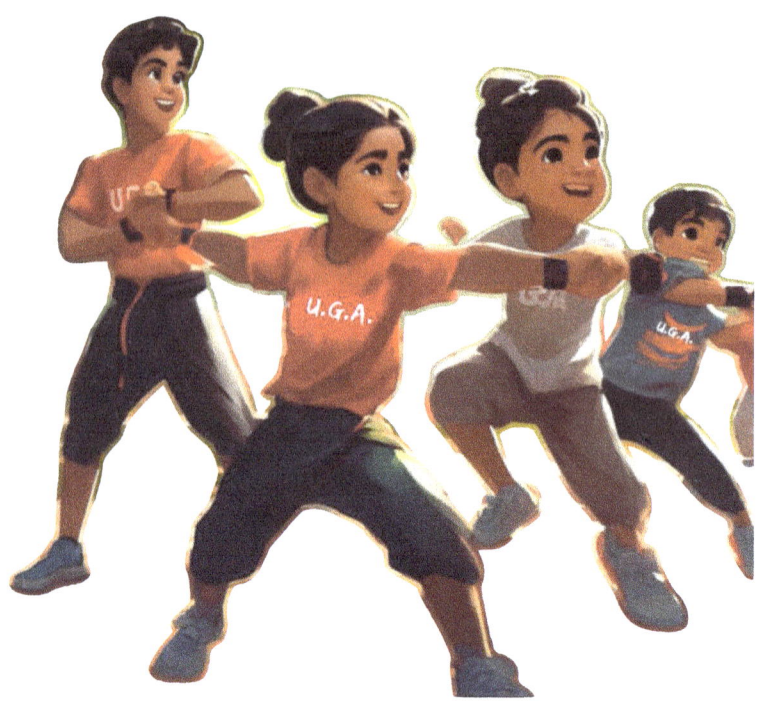

Training at Any Age:

At the Universal Grappling Academy, we start training kids from the age of 4. If you get them started early when their brains are like sponges, they'll soak up more of the information that your training routines provide. They'll be more ready for competition (if that's what they want to do) in a year or two once they are settled into a daily training regimen. Like school, it should be a part of their daily routine that isn't an option.

What does training do for the kids at an early age? It teaches them self-defense, confidence, focus, routine, discipline, a healthy lifestyle, teamwork, persistence, and perseverance.

Training at the Universal Grappling Academy can provide numerous benefits for children. Here are some reasons to sign them up and/or keep them involved.

1. Physical Fitness: Grappling and Striking training promote overall physical health, helping children develop strength, flexibility, and endurance while combating childhood obesity.

2. Self-Defense Skills: Learning striking and grappling techniques equips children with essential self-defense skills, boosting their confidence and ability to protect themselves if necessary.

3. Discipline and Focus: Regular training fosters discipline and focus as children learn to follow instructions, set goals, and work towards improvement, which can translate into better combat sports and academic performance.

4. Social Skills: Training in a team environment encourages teamwork, communication, and respect for others, helping children build strong social connections and friendships.

5. Confidence Building: As children progress in their skills and mastery of techniques, they gain self-esteem and confidence, which can positively impact various aspects of their lives. Not only will they have the confidence to stand up for themselves, but they'll also have the skills..

6. Emotional Resilience: Grappling teaches children how to handle challenges, setbacks, and competition, fostering resilience and a positive mindset in overcoming obstacles.

7. Healthy Lifestyle Habits: Exposure to martial arts can instill lifelong habits of physical activity and healthy living, promoting a balanced lifestyle as they grow.

8. Stress Relief: Physical activity is a great way to manage stress and anxiety. UGA-MMA provides an outlet for children to release energy and emotions in a constructive manner.

9. Goal Setting and Achievement: MMA training allows children to set personal goals, whether it's earning a new belt or mastering a technique, teaching them about perseverance and the rewards of hard work. They'll learn that Hard Work Pays Off.

10. Fun and Engagement: UGA-MMA is an exciting and dynamic program that keeps children engaged and motivated, making exercise enjoyable rather than a chore.

Overall, training at the Universal Grappling Academy can provide children with a well-rounded experience that supports their physical, mental, and emotional development. Your kids can literally grow up training at the UGA and can become Combat Sports Regional, National, or World Champions, as many have done.

The mid to older generations that want to train and possibly compete start from the upper teen years to able-bodied senior citizens. If you live and train properly, you can enjoy a healthy and physical life from beginning to end.

The same benefits that nurture the children will also benefit the teens and adults. There isn't an age limit to training if you take care of yourself and respect your limitations. Age is Just a Number. Remember, not everyone wants to or can compete, but for those who can and want to, stick to the path and trust the UGA process.

What you'll need:
- Proper Training - At a UGA International Facility.
- Proper Conditioning - Cardio, Speed, Agility, Flexibility.
- Proper Nutrition - Eating Right and Efficient Hydration
- Proper Recovery - Rest and Healing.
- Proper Mental State - Stay Strong, Focused & Ready.
- Proper Attitude - Stay Humble and Focused.
- Proper Support - Family, Friends, and Teammates.

Basic Fundamentals of MMA

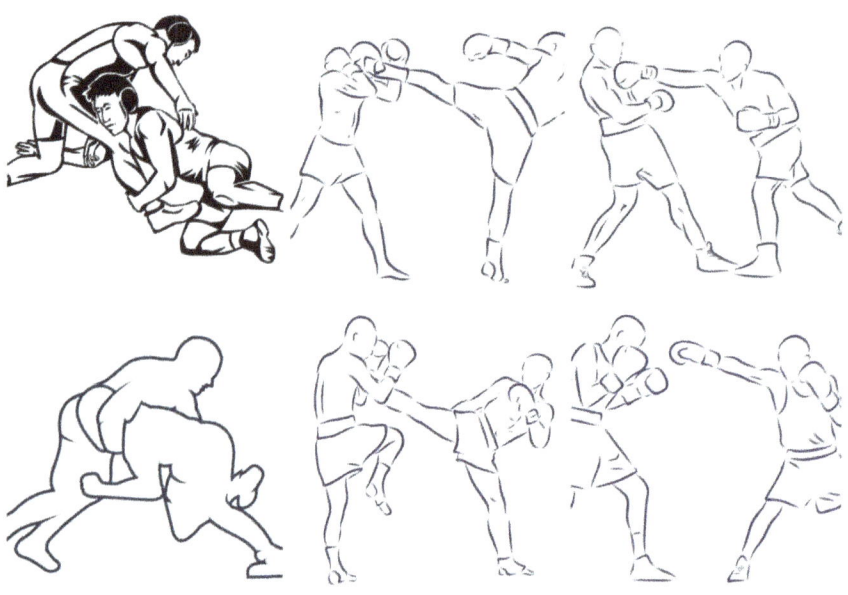

Here's a look into the fundamentals of MMA, focusing on basic striking techniques and grappling.

Striking Techniques

1. Punches:
  - *Jab:* This should be fast and accurate. A quick, straight punch thrown with the lead hand; used for distance management and setting up combinations.
  - *Cross:* A powerful straight punch thrown with the rear hand; often follows a jab and can be used to capitalize on openings.
  - *Hook:* A punch that comes from the side, targeting the opponent's head or body; effective at close range.
  - *Uppercut:* An upward punch aimed at the opponent's chin; useful for countering an opponent's guard and creating openings.

2. Kicks:
  - *Push Kicks:* A straight kick delivered with the ball or heel of the foot; can be used to maintain distance or as a quick strike.
  - *Roundhouse Kick:* A powerful kick delivered by striking with preferably with the shin bone rather than the foot, coming from the side; targets the legs, body, or head.
  - *Side Kick:* A kick delivered by turning the body and striking with the heel or blade of the foot; effective for maintaining distance.
  - *Back Kick:* A kick delivered by thrusting the heel back towards an opponent; useful for countering aggressive forward movement.

3. Elbows:
- *Horizontal Elbow:* A sideways strike that can be used in close range, effective for cutting and damaging.
- *Diagonal Elbow:* Thrown at an angle, targeting the opponent's head; useful in clinch situations.
- *Back Elbow:* A reverse strike delivered while turning away from an opponent; effective when exiting from a clinch.

4. Knees:
- *Standing Knee:* A strike delivered by driving the knee through their opponent and not up to them, often used in clinch situations.
- *Jumping Knee:* A powerful knee strike executed while jumping; can catch opponents off-guard, especially when they are moving in.

Grappling Techniques

1. Takedowns:
- *Single Leg Takedown:* A technique where the fighter grabs one of the opponent's legs and uses leverage to bring them to the ground.
- *Double Leg Takedown:* A more powerful takedown that involves grabbing both legs of the opponent and driving forward to take them down.
- *Body Lock Takedown:* Involves wrapping the arms around the opponent's body and using momentum to bring them to the ground.

2. Throws:
- *Hip Throw (O Goshi):* A technique borrowed from judo where the fighter uses their hip as a pivot point to throw the opponent over.
- *Shoulder Throw (Seoi Nage):* Another judo technique that involves using the shoulder to lift and throw the opponent.
- *Fireman's Carry:* A wrestling takedown that involves lifting the opponent over the shoulder and bringing them to the ground.

3. Holds:
- *Guards:* Positions where one fighter is on their back with their legs wrapped around the opponent; includes open guard, closed guard, butterfly guard, and half guard.
- *Side Control:* A dominant position where one fighter is lying perpendicular to the opponent, controlling their upper body.
- *Mount:* A dominant position where one fighter sits on top of the opponent's torso, offering the ability to strike or use submission moves.

Understanding these fundamentals is crucial for students looking to train in MMA. They form the foundation for advanced techniques and strategies in the sport.

Understanding Competition Rules

It's important to educate yourself about your sport and know the Rules and Regulations for a Grappling Tournament or MMA Fight. You need to know what moves are legal or illegal during the match and how you can use them to your advantage in the process of winning your competition.

   - Weight Classes - Weight classes and the rules in a grappling tournament vary by organization. Weight classes for MMA are now uniform. Know what class you'll perform your best in and train close to the top of that weight class for your best opportunity for success.

Weight classes in pounds:

115 - Atom weight (women)
125 - Fly weight (men & women)
135 - Bantamweight (men & women)
145 - Featherweight (men & women)
155 - Lightweight (men & Women)
170 - Welterweight (men)
185 - Middleweight (men)
205 - Light Heavyweight (men)
206 - 265 - Heavyweight (men)
266+ - Super Heavyweight (men)

   - Scoring and Judging in MMA - Grappling tournaments vary depending on what moves they'll score. I believe that all tournaments should have a uniform code of moves and points so as not to have to figure out what's legal or how to get the most points from tournament to tournament. We train our UGA grappling competitors that being aggressive and getting the initial takedown and control position (full mount/side mount/back mount) is the best way to get your points, and then going for your submission moves. Other schools will teach their kids to get some points and then stall out with a guard or mount for the remaining time. This isn't grappling, and we definitely want our UGA kids/adults to be more active.

In an MMA bout, I will give some basic rules on how to win your fight. One of the number one things I like to drive into my students is that you need to control the outcome of your fight (Win your fight by knockout / TKO / or Submission)because, if you leave it to the judges, then you aren't in control of the outcome.

Basic Rules for MMA

1. Weight Classes: Fighters are categorized into weight classes to ensure a fair match.

2. Prohibited Actions (Fouls):
No groin attacks: No striking, kicking, grabbing, or any other action targeting the groin area.

No attacks to the head/spine/neck: No strikes, knees, or kicks to the back of the head, the spine, or the throat.
No eye gouging: No intentional eye gouging or manipulation of the fingers.
No grabbing or biting: No grabbing of the throat, clothes, hair pulling, or biting of an opponent.
No head-butts: No intentional head-butts or use of the head as a striking instrument.
No fish hooking or grabbing: No fish hooking or intentional grabbing of the ring or cage.
No excessive language: Abusive language is prohibited, and the referee decides if language crosses the line.
No striking of a grounded opponent: Fighters are prohibited from striking a grounded opponent using knees or kicks to the head.

Approved Techniques:

Striking:
Fighters can use a variety of striking techniques, including punches, kicks, and elbows, to attack their opponent.
Grappling:
Fighters can attempt to take their opponent down and control them on the ground using grappling techniques.
Submissions:
Fighters can submit their opponent by applying various joint locks or chokes.

Ending A Fight

Knockout (KO): A fighter loses consciousness or is incapacitated due to legal strikes.
Technical Knockout (TKO): A fight is stopped if a fighter is unable to continue due to injuries or the referee deems them unable to fight.
Submission: A fighter taps out or verbally concedes to a submission hold.
Referee Stoppage: The referee can stop the fight if they believe one fighter is unable to continue due to injury or is no longer able to defend themselves.
Decision: If the fight reaches the round limit, the bout is scored by judges, and a winner is declared based on the points.

Other Important Rules:

Equipment:
Fighters are required to wear approved shorts, gloves, mouth guards, and groin protection.
Rounds:
MMA fights are typically divided into rounds with a set duration.
Amateur - 3x2 minute rounds or 3x3 minute rounds
Pro - 3x5 minute rounds or 5x5 minute rounds

Judging:
Bouts are evaluated and scored by three judges using the 10-Point Must System.

Sports Conditioning for MMA

- Importance of Conditioning in MMA - "Fatigue Makes Cowards Out of All Men/Women". If you can't breathe, you can't fight, no matter how good you are.

Conditioning is a crucial aspect of UGA mixed martial arts training for several reasons:

1. Endurance: MMA fights can be physically demanding, often lasting several rounds. Proper conditioning enhances cardiovascular endurance, allowing fighters to maintain high levels of performance throughout the fight without succumbing to fatigue. It's important that a UGA fighter needs to be able to out-move, out-work, and outlast their opponent.

2. Strength: Conditioning includes strength training, which is vital for grappling, striking, and overall combat effectiveness. Increased strength helps fighters execute techniques more effectively and resist opponents' attacks.

3. Speed and Agility: Effective conditioning improves a fighter's speed, agility, and reaction times. This is essential for dodging strikes, closing distance quickly, and executing techniques seamlessly.

4. Recovery: Good conditioning allows fighters to recover more quickly between rounds and after intense training sessions. This means they can train harder and more frequently, leading to better overall performance.

5. Mental Toughness: Conditioning not only improves physical capabilities but also builds mental resilience. Pushing through tough conditioning workouts helps fighters develop the mindset needed to face the challenges of competition.

6. Injury Prevention: A well-conditioned athlete is less prone to injuries. Stronger muscles and joints can withstand the rigors of training and competition, reducing the risk of strains and sprains.

7. Weight Management: Conditioning routines, particularly those that include high-intensity interval training (HIIT), can help fighters maintain or reach their desired weight class more effectively.

Flexibility and Mobility Training

- Importance of Flexibility in MMA - The more flexible that you are, the easier it is to avoid not only submission attempts, but also injuries during training.

Flexibility and mobility play essential roles in UGA mixed martial arts training and competition.

1. Injury Prevention: Improved flexibility and mobility help reduce the risk of injuries by allowing the body to move through its full range of motion without strain. This is crucial in a sport where the body is subjected to various stresses and impacts.

2. Technique Execution: Many MMA techniques, such as kicks, submissions, and grappling maneuvers, require a high degree of flexibility and mobility. Enhanced flexibility helps athletes execute these techniques more effectively and with greater precision.

3. Range of Motion: Greater flexibility allows fighters to move more freely, making it easier to evade strikes, change angles, and engage in various positions during grappling exchanges. This adaptability can be a significant advantage in a fight.

4. Balance and Stability: Flexibility contributes to better balance and stability, which are crucial for maintaining control during striking and grappling. A flexible fighter can adjust their body position quickly, enhancing their ability to stay on their feet or maintain dominant positions on the ground.

5. Recovery: Flexibility and mobility exercises can aid in recovery after intense training sessions or fights. Stretching and mobility work can help alleviate muscle tension and soreness, promoting faster recovery and readiness for subsequent workouts.

6. Performance Enhancement: Increased flexibility and mobility can improve overall athletic performance. Fighters who can move fluidly and efficiently are often better equipped to execute complex techniques and adapt to their opponents' movements.

7. Mental Focus: Engaging in flexibility and mobility training can also enhance mental focus and body awareness. This mindfulness can be beneficial during fights, as it allows athletes to stay in tune with their bodies and make quick adjustments.

In summary, flexibility and mobility are vital components of an MMA fighter's training regimen, impacting their overall performance, injury prevention, and ability to execute techniques effectively.

Nutrition for MMA Performance

Nutrition plays a critical role in the success of UGA Combat Sports Competitors.

1. Performance Optimization: Proper nutrition fuels the body, providing the necessary energy for intense training sessions and fights. A well-balanced diet ensures fighters have the stamina and strength to perform at their best.

2. Weight Management: Many fighters need to maintain or reach specific weight classes. Nutrition helps regulate body composition, allowing athletes to manage weight effectively while preserving muscle mass and minimizing fat.

3. Recovery: Nutrition is essential for recovery after workouts and fights. Consuming the right nutrients, such as proteins, carbohydrates, and healthy fats, aids in muscle repair, reduces soreness, and replenishes glycogen stores.

4. Injury Prevention: A balanced diet rich in vitamins and minerals supports overall health and helps strengthen bones, muscles, and connective tissues. This can reduce the risk of injuries during training and competition.

5. Mental Focus: Nutrition impacts cognitive function and mental clarity. A well-nourished brain can enhance concentration, decision-making, and reaction times during fights, which are crucial for success in the cage.

6. Hydration: Proper hydration is a vital aspect of nutrition. Staying hydrated helps maintain optimal physical performance, regulates body temperature, and supports overall health. Dehydration can lead to fatigue, decreased endurance, and increased risk of injury.

7. Adaptation to Training: Nutrition supports the body's adaptation to the physical demands of MMA training. Adequate intake of macronutrients helps improve strength, endurance, and overall athletic performance.

8. Long-term Health: A nutritious diet contributes to long-term health and well-being, reducing the risk of chronic diseases and ensuring that fighters can continue to train and compete effectively throughout their careers.

Remember, proper nutrition is fundamental for UGA MMA competitors, impacting their performance, recovery, weight management, and overall health, ultimately contributing to their success in the sport.

Pre-Fight Nutrition Strategy

A well-planned pre-fight nutrition strategy is crucial for UGA MMA Combat Sports Team Competitors to optimize performance, enhance energy levels, and ensure proper recovery.

1. Timing
- *Days Leading Up to the Fight:* Focus on a balanced diet rich in carbohydrates, proteins, and healthy fats. Aim to maintain hydration and avoid drastic weight cuts.
- *24-48 Hours Before the Fight:* Start tapering your food intake to lighter meals that are easy to digest. Increase carbohydrate intake to maximize glycogen stores.

2. Macronutrient Focus
- *Carbohydrates:*
  - *Sources:* Rice, pasta, quinoa, sweet potatoes, fruits.
  - *Goal:* Consume complex carbohydrates to ensure glycogen stores are full. Aim for 60-70% of total caloric intake from carbohydrates in the days leading up to the fight.

- *Proteins:*
  - *Sources:* Lean meats (chicken, turkey, fish), eggs, dairy, legumes.
  - *Goal:* Maintain muscle mass and support recovery. Aim for moderate protein intake (about 20-30% of total caloric intake).

- *Fats:*
  - *Sources:* Avocados, nuts, seeds, olive oil.
  - *Goal:* Include healthy fats in moderation (about 10-20% of total caloric intake) for energy and overall health.

3. Hydration
- *Days Before the Fight:* Drink plenty of water throughout the days leading up to the fight. Aim for at least half your body weight in ounces of water daily.
- *24 Hours Before:* Increase electrolyte intake (sodium, potassium) through foods or sports drinks to maintain fluid balance and prevent dehydration.

4. Pre-Fight Meal
- *Timing:* 3-4 hours before the fight.
- *Meal Composition:*
  - *Carbohydrates:* Focus on easily digestible carbs (e.g., oatmeal, rice, bananas).
  - *Proteins:* Include a small portion of lean protein (e.g., chicken, turkey, or a protein shake).
  - *Fats:* Keep fats minimal to prevent gastrointestinal discomfort.
- *Example Meal:*
  - Grilled chicken breast with white rice and steamed vegetables (carrots, zucchini) or a banana with a scoop of protein powder mixed with water.

5. Snacks
- *1-2 Hours Before the Fight:* If needed, consume a light snack that is high in carbohydrates and low in protein and fat to avoid feeling heavy.
- *Snack Options:*
  - Energy bar, banana, or a small serving of applesauce.

6. Mental Preparation
- *Stay Calm:* Maintain a calm mindset during the pre-fight period. Avoid trying new foods to prevent any digestive issues.
- *Visualize Success:* Along with nutrition, focus on mental strategies to boost confidence and concentration.

7. Post-Fight Recovery
- After the fight, prioritize rehydration and a balanced meal to aid recovery. Include carbohydrates for glycogen replenishment, protein for muscle recovery, and healthy fats.

This pre-fight nutrition strategy aims to maximize energy levels, maintain hydration, and support optimal performance during the fight. Tailoring the specifics to individual preferences and dietary restrictions is essential for the best results.

Resistance Training for Competition

Resistance training is a crucial component for UGA fighters and grappling tournament competitors, as it enhances their overall performance and reduces the risk of injury.

1. Increased Strength: Resistance training builds muscle strength, which is vital for grapplers and fighters who rely on explosive power during takedowns, submissions, and striking. Stronger muscles can generate more force, leading to improved performance in matches.

2. Improved Endurance: Incorporating resistance training into their regimen can enhance muscular endurance, allowing athletes to maintain their strength and performance levels throughout the duration of a fight or match, which is especially important in grappling, where matches can be prolonged.

3. Enhanced Stability and Balance: Many resistance training exercises improve core stability and balance, which are essential for maintaining control during grappling exchanges and striking. A strong core helps fighters absorb impacts and maintain proper posture.

4. Injury Prevention: Targeted resistance training can help strengthen ligaments and tendons, which may reduce the likelihood of injuries. Stronger muscles provide better support for joints, which is crucial in high-contact sports.

5. Functional Movement: Resistance training can be designed to mimic the movements performed in fighting and grappling, enhancing the UGA athlete's ability to execute techniques effectively. Exercises that focus on functional strength translate directly to performance in the ring or on the mat.

6. Psychological Benefits: Regular training can boost confidence and mental resilience. Knowing that they are physically prepared can help fighters maintain composure and focus during competition. Strength = Confidence.

7. Weight Management: For fighters who need to maintain a specific weight class, resistance training helps build lean muscle mass while also promoting fat loss and aiding in effective weight management.

Plyometric Workout for UGA Competitors

A plyometric routine can greatly enhance explosiveness, agility, and overall athletic performance for UGA MMA fighters and grappling competitors.

Warm-Up (10-15 minutes)
- Dynamic stretches (leg swings, arm circles, torso twists)
- Light jogging or skipping
- Mobility drills focusing on hips, shoulders, and ankles

Plyometric Exercises (3-4 sets of each exercise with 30-60 seconds rest between sets)

1. Box Jumps
  - *Reps:* 8-10
  - Focus on jumping explosively onto a sturdy box or platform. Step down and repeat.

2. Depth Jumps
  - *Reps:* 6-8
  - Step off a box (12-24 inches) and upon landing, jump vertically as high as possible.

3. Burpee Tuck Jumps
  - *Reps:* 6-10
  - Perform a burpee, and as you jump back up, tuck your knees towards your chest.

4. Lateral Bounds
  - Reps: 8-10 per side
  - Jump sideways from one leg to the other, focusing on distance and quick landings.

5. Single-Leg Hops
  - *Reps:* 6-8 per leg
  - Hop forward on one leg for distance, focusing on balance and control during landing.

6. Clap Push-Ups
  - *Reps:* 6-10
  - Perform a push-up, but push off explosively to clap your hands before landing back down.

7. Medicine Ball Slams
  - *Reps:* 10-12
  - Use a medicine ball to slam down to the ground with maximum force, focusing on your core and leg engagement.

Cool Down (10 minutes)
- Static stretching focusing on legs, back, and shoulders
- Deep breathing exercises to promote recovery

Additional Tips:
- *Form First:* Prioritize proper technique over speed to prevent injury.
- *Progress Gradually:* Increase intensity or volume as strength and explosiveness improve.
- *Incorporate into Regular Training:* Combine plyometrics with other strength and skill training for a well-rounded approach.
- *Listen to Your Body:* Adequate rest and recovery are essential, especially with high-impact exercises.

This routine will not only build explosive power but also improve agility and coordination, which are key attributes for success in UGA MMA and grappling competitions.

Endurance Training is an important Step to Winning

I always like to emphasize that a strong endurance program is key to you out-moving, out-working, and out-lasting your opponents in a grappling tournament or MMA fight. When you push your opponents to their limits (as we all have them), they'll lose breath, speed, strength, and confidence. At that point, they'll go from the angry and aggressive bull competing to win to now competing just to survive! If you can push your opponents past their conditioning limits, you'll push them into defeat.

At the Universal Grappling Academy, we use a wide variety of training tools to work on and improve our endurance.

Short / Long Blocks - 1/2 Mile to 1 Mile plus distance running.
Stop Signs - A quarter-mile sprint from stop sign to stop sign.
Sled Pulls - Sprint Pulling a weighted sled 25-50 yards.
Wheelbarrow Pushes - A weighted wheelbarrow run.
Sprints - 50 - 100 yard sprint. There and back.
Treadmill to Cross Trainer - 60-second intervals.
Running Lines / Suicides - 3 sets of fast runs.
Kettle Bell Runs - sprint with Kettle Bells one way and sprint back without them, then go in reverse.
Intense Striking or Grappling Drills - 30-60-90 second non-stop functional movements consisting of striking and or grappling drills.

Mental Conditioning and Focus for Competitions

Mental conditioning and focus are crucial elements in the preparation and performance of competitors in MMA and grappling. The psychological aspect of sports can often be as important as physical training, influencing an athlete's ability to perform under pressure, manage stress, and maintain peak performance.

Importance of Mental Conditioning and Focus

1. Stress Management: High-pressure situations, such as competitions, can induce anxiety. Mental conditioning helps athletes develop coping strategies to manage stress and remain calm during a match.

2. Enhanced Concentration: Maintaining focus on the task at hand is vital in combat sports, where distractions can lead to mistakes. Mental conditioning helps sharpen concentration and reduces the likelihood of lapses in focus.

3. Improved Confidence: A strong mental game boosts self-belief. Competitors who engage in mental conditioning often visualize success and reinforce positive self-talk, which enhances their confidence.

4. Resilience: The ability to bounce back from setbacks is essential in sports. Mental conditioning fosters resilience, allowing athletes to learn from losses and maintain a positive mindset.
5. Strategic Thinking: Competitors need to adapt quickly during matches. Mental training helps develop strategic thinking and the ability to read opponents, making quick decisions based on situational awareness.

Techniques Used by Competitors for Mental Conditioning

1. Visualization: Athletes often use visualization techniques to mentally rehearse their performance. This may involve imagining themselves executing techniques successfully, overcoming challenges, or winning matches.

2. Meditation and Mindfulness: Many athletes practice meditation or mindfulness to improve focus and reduce anxiety. These practices help create a calm mind, allowing competitors to stay present and focused during competitions.

3. Goal Setting: Establishing clear, achievable goals helps athletes maintain motivation and direction. Competitors often set both short-term and long-term goals to track their progress and stay focused on their objectives.

4. Positive Self-Talk: Developing a habit of positive affirmations and self-talk can counter negative thoughts and build confidence. Competitors may use mantras or phrases to keep themselves motivated and focused.

5. Mental Rehearsal: This involves mentally going through the motions of a fight or match repeatedly, which can enhance muscle memory and reduce anxiety about performance.

6. Breathing Techniques: Competitors use controlled breathing exercises to manage stress and maintain focus. Deep breathing can help lower heart rates and promote relaxation before and during competitions.

7. Working with Sports Psychologists: Many athletes collaborate with sports psychologists who provide tailored mental conditioning programs, helping them develop strategies specific to their needs and challenges.

8. Routine Development: Establishing pre-fight routines can help competitors get into the right mental state. This could include specific warm-ups, visualization, or rituals that create a sense of familiarity and comfort.

The combination of physical prowess and mental strength is key to success in MMA and grappling.

The Importance of Sparring and Live Combat Drills

Sparring and live combat drills are essential components of training at the Universal Grappling Academy (UGA). These methods provide numerous benefits that contribute to the overall development of UGA fighters and grapplers.

Importance of Sparring
1. Realistic Application: Sparring allows athletes to practice techniques in a realistic and dynamic environment. This helps them understand how techniques work under pressure and against resisting opponents.

2. Timing and Distance Control: Sparring helps competitors develop a sense of timing and distance, which are crucial for effective striking and grappling. Athletes learn to gauge when to attack, defend, or escape.

3. Adaptability: Engaging in sparring sessions exposes fighters to various styles and strategies. This variability forces them to adapt and develop a more versatile skill set, improving their overall game.

4. Pressure Management: Sparring simulates the pressure of competition, helping athletes manage anxiety and stress. Practicing under these conditions prepares them for the mental challenges faced during actual fights.

5. Feedback and Improvement: Sparring provides immediate feedback on techniques and strategies. Athletes can identify strengths and weaknesses, allowing them to refine their skills and address gaps in their training.

6. Building Endurance: Sparring is physically demanding, helping athletes build cardiovascular endurance and muscular stamina. This conditioning is vital for performing at high levels throughout a match or fight.

Importance of Live Combat Drills

1. Specific Skill Development: Live combat drills focus on particular techniques or scenarios, allowing athletes to hone specific skills in a controlled environment. This targeted practice can lead to quicker improvements.

2. Problem-Solving: These drills encourage fighters to think critically and solve problems in real-time, enhancing their decision-making abilities. They learn to respond effectively to an opponent's actions.

3. Collaboration: Live combat drills often involve partners working together to simulate match conditions. This collaboration fosters a sense of community and teamwork, essential in any training environment.

4. Injury Prevention: Practicing techniques in a controlled, live setting allows athletes to learn proper mechanics and body movements, reducing the risk of injury during actual competition.

5. Integration of Techniques: Live drills help athletes integrate various techniques into their game, allowing them to transition smoothly between striking, grappling, and defensive maneuvers.

6. Confidence Building: Regular practice in live drills builds confidence in an athlete's skills and abilities. Knowing they can apply techniques effectively in a dynamic environment boosts self-esteem.

Conclusion

Both sparring and live combat drills play a pivotal role in the training regimen at the UGA. They provide athletes with the opportunity to apply their skills in realistic settings, develop adaptability, and enhance their overall performance. By incorporating these practices into their training, competitors can better prepare for the challenges of competition, ultimately leading to improved outcomes in their fighting and grappling careers.

**When it's Time to Fight,
Don't fight, Afraid, Don't fight to Survive, Fight to Win!**

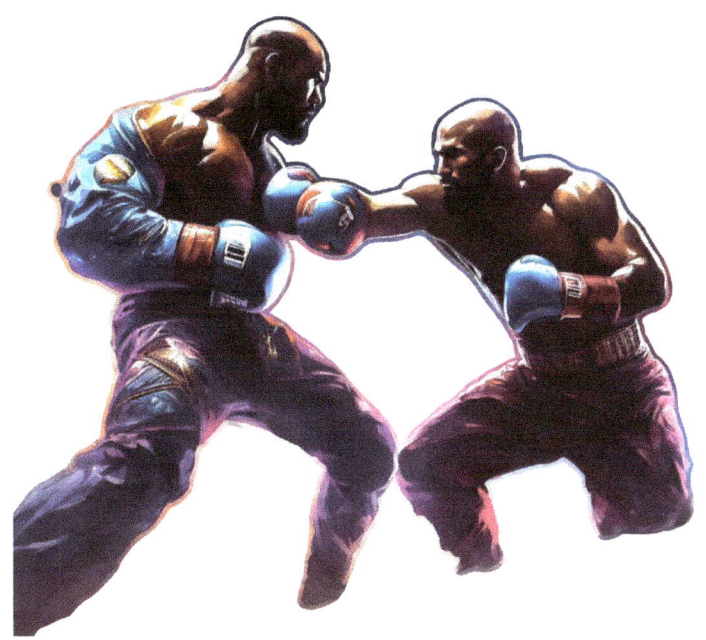

CHAPTER 8

SAFETY AND AWARENESS

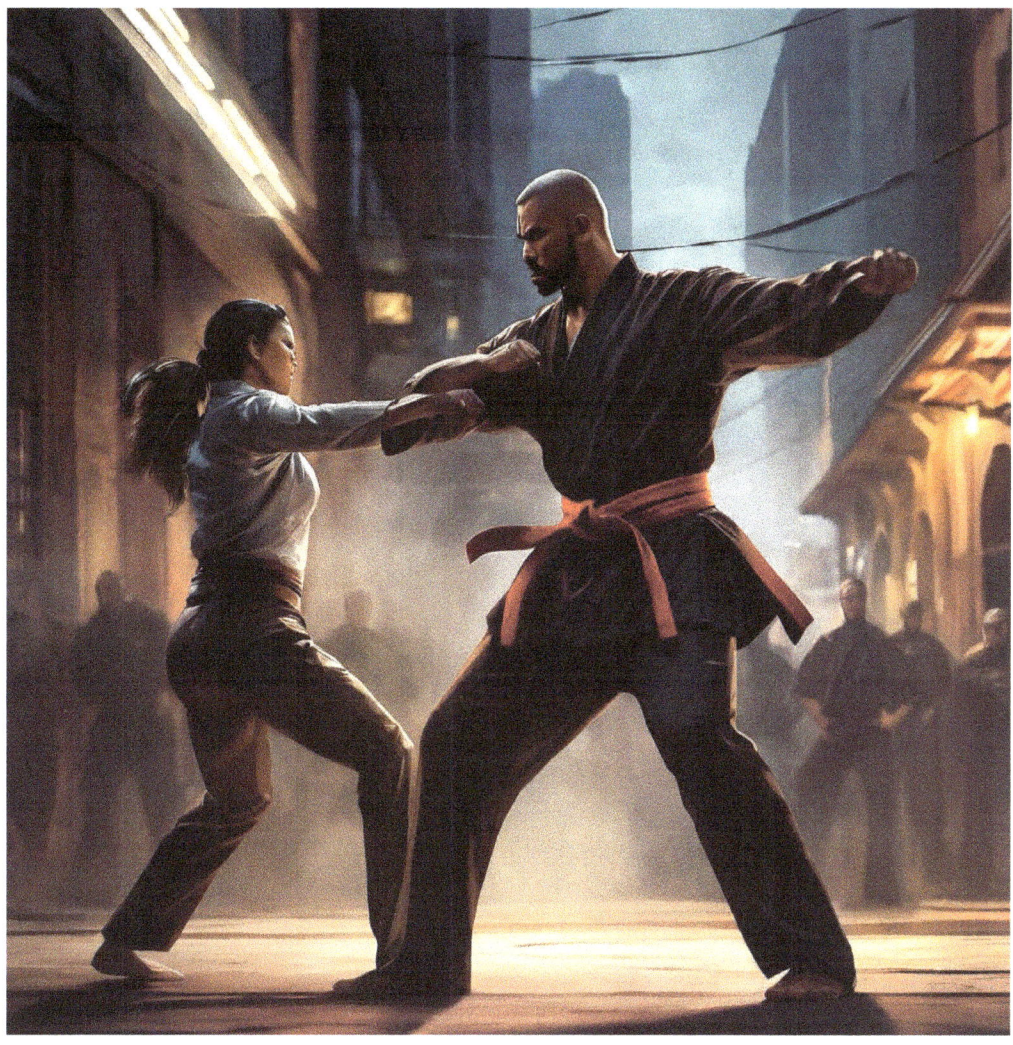

Keeping yourself safe by being aware of your surroundings and the actions happening around you is important and a major part of learning UGA Mixed Martial Arts for Self Defense. Whether you're here to protect and defend yourself or somebody else, being aware of the people and situations around you is paramount.

Safety and Awareness By Coach Tyson Johnson
Tips and Suggestions to help keep you safe in today`s unsafe world
" It`s Better to be Prepared than to Be a Victim"

➢ Personal safety begins with an individual's awareness of their environment – no one can defend against danger they don't see coming. Taking your safety seriously doesn't just help you, but can help your family, friends and benefit others as well.

➢ Set the home address in your smartphone, GPS, and other devices to an address near your home, but not to your actual home address.

➢ Keep your key fob or physical car key in your hand when walking alone, especially in parking lots. If possible, leave with others out the doors when shopping.

➤ Do not overshare on social media. Don't give your personal information (D.O.B. / SSN).

➤ Don't give money to beggars in a parking lot – No Matter what sob story they may give you about them, their broken down vehicle or their kids.

➤ When leaving any store, scan the parking lot, don't be on your phone or distracted, keep an eye out for strangers loitering in the parking lot or watching you.

➤ If sitting in your vehicle, keep your doors locked and windows only partially down. Be aware of strangers approaching you or your vehicle in a parking lot. Distraction scams are a sure way to become a victim.

➤ Keep your keys on you and lock your doors when getting gas. Keep an eye out for people approaching you, this is a good way to distract you or find out if you have cash!

➤ Be sure to lock the doors of your vehicle when leaving it and always look in the back seats floor area before getting in.

➤ When fueling your vehicle, check for information skimmers and hidden cameras.

➤ Don't fall for fake phone calls or emails. Never give your personal information to id yourself unless you are sure the company is legitimate.

➤ Always be aware of your exits, and have an exit strategy. Practice devising alternate methods of escape if your primary exit becomes compromised.

➤ Utilize walls and other barriers to protect your back and sides and maximize your field of vision, taking care not to back yourself into a corner. Practice this in public places, such as seating in restaurants, waiting rooms, or shopping centers.

➤ One of your biggest advantages in a dangerous situation is being able to see the danger coming with enough time to react appropriately. When your range of vision is limited, get creative about ways to expand it and give yourself an advantage – practice utilizing store windows, car windshields, or even other people's sunglasses to detect threats you wouldn't be able to see otherwise.

➤ If you feel like you are being followed, either on foot or in a vehicle, stop and turn around, pretending as if you went the wrong way. The reaction of the person following you will help you determine if they are indeed a threat: If they stop or reroute to mirror your actions, then you can confirm that they are following you intentionally.

➤ Those with malicious intent generally single out individuals that seem meek, vulnerable, or unaware of their surroundings. At the UGA we teach that body language plays a confidence, awareness, and capability role; regardless of how you actually feel, can help broadcast to any threats that you are an undesirable target, and increase your personal safety.

➢ If someone is crowding you, seems suspicious, or is displaying threatening body language, scan them for subtle signs of violent intent or a hidden weapon. Increase the distance between yourself and this person – the amount of distance depends on the situation, but five or six feet can allow you some reaction time if they become an active threat.

➢ Trust your gut. If you get the sense that something is wrong or doesn't add up, do not ignore it. Your instincts exist to protect you – it is always better to be overcautious than to ignore warning signs that turned out to be legitimate.

➢ Be sure to watch your garage door close completely to avoid someone slipping in underneath it as you walk inside.

➢ Learn and practice UGA Self Defense skills. Make sure you are in good enough condition to defend yourself and your family in a combat situation.

➢ Just because somebody looks nice, doesn't mean that they are nice. Good strangers look just like bad strangers.

➢ If a stranger tries to grab you, scream at the top of your lungs "Stop Touching Me or Fire". You should also hit, kick, claw and do anything you can to escape their grasp.

➢ If a stranger tries to approach you in their car, stay away from the vehicle and start walking in the opposite direction. Use your phone and start recording them if they don't leave you alone immediately.

➢ If a stranger attempts to approach you and you are uncomfortable, stay away and try to move in to where there is a crowd of people, there is safety in numbers and it'll be hard for them to do anything.

➢ Kids don't talk to strangers, don't allow them to lure you in to their traps, don't give them your name or information in person or on the phone, don't open a door to a stranger or tell anybody where you live, don't give your information on social media/game programs or anywhere else.

There are many ways to keep yourself and your family safe, I hope this will help give you some knowledge on how to prevent yourselves from becoming victims.

Why Training Children is Important

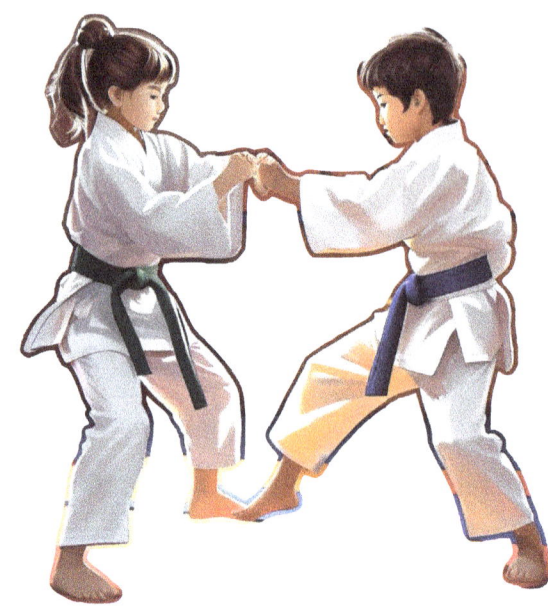

Training children from 4 to 17 years old in Mixed Martial Arms (MMA), Self Defense, and Sports Conditioning at the Universal Grappling Academy (UGA) is crucial to their development: We help them expand their knowledge and build Combat Sports skills that'll benefit them in competition or for self defense now and in the future.

1. Bully Prevention: Teaching children effective self-defense techniques empowers them to handle bullying situations confidently. They learn not only how to protect themselves but also how to avoid and de-escalate conflicts.

2. Self-Confidence: As children progress through training and master new skills, their self-esteem grows. This enhanced confidence can positively impact their academic performance and social interactions.

3. Discipline: Learning martial arts requires focus, commitment, and the ability to follow instructions. These qualities foster self-discipline, which is beneficial both in and out of the training environment.

4. Team Building: Participating in group classes encourages teamwork and camaraderie. Children learn to support one another, leading to stronger friendships and social skills.

5. Self-Defense: Understanding self-defense techniques equips children with the knowledge to protect themselves in dangerous situations, promoting a sense of safety and security.

6. Structure and Respect: The structured environment of martial arts training teaches children respect for their instructors, peers, and themselves. This respect translates into their interactions in everyday life.

7. Honor: Instilling a sense of honor encourages children to act with integrity and uphold ethical standards, both on and off the mat.

8. Mental, Physical, and Emotional Strength: Training develops not only physical fitness but also mental resilience and emotional intelligence. Children learn to cope with challenges, manage stress, and develop a strong mindset.

Overall, the holistic approach of the UGA ensures that children are not just learning martial arts techniques but are also developing essential life skills that will serve them well into adulthood.

Why Training Law Enforcement is Important

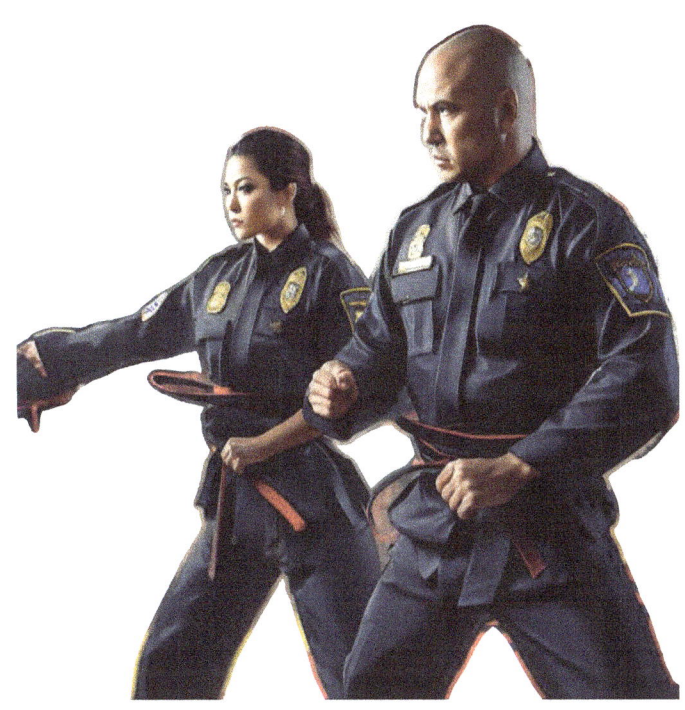

Training law enforcement in Mixed Martial Arts (MMA), Self Defense, and Conditioning at the Universal Grappling Academy (UGA) is vital for our community.

1. Hand-to-Hand Combat Skills: In situations where officers may need to engage in close-quarters combat, having strong hand-to-hand combat skills is essential for their safety and that of the public. Effective techniques can help them control situations without excessive force.

2. Self-Confidence While on Duty: Training builds confidence in officers 'abilities to handle various scenarios. This self-assurance can improve decision-making under pressure, allowing them to respond effectively to threats.

3. Self-Defense: Law enforcement officers often face unpredictable and potentially violent encounters. Training in self-defense equips them with the skills needed to protect themselves and de-escalate situations effectively.

4. Understanding Criminal Mindsets: As criminals increasingly train in combat sports, law enforcement must be prepared to face adversaries who are physically skilled. By training in UGA-MMA, officers can better anticipate and counter these tactics.

5. Use of Force Training: Integrating UGA-MMA and self-defense training helps officers understand the appropriate levels of force to apply in various scenarios. This knowledge is crucial for making informed, ethical decisions during encounters.

6. Mental, Physical, and Emotional Strength: The rigorous training regimen enhances officers' physical fitness, mental resilience, and emotional stability. This comprehensive approach prepares them to handle the stresses of the job and maintain composure in challenging situations.

7. Community Trust and Safety: Well-trained officers can navigate conflicts more effectively, leading to reduced incidents of excessive force and improved community relations. This fosters trust between law enforcement and the communities they serve.

Overall, the training provided at UGA not only equips law enforcement with practical skills but also promotes a positive approach to their well-being and effectiveness, ultimately benefiting both the officers and the communities they protect.

Why Training Women is Important

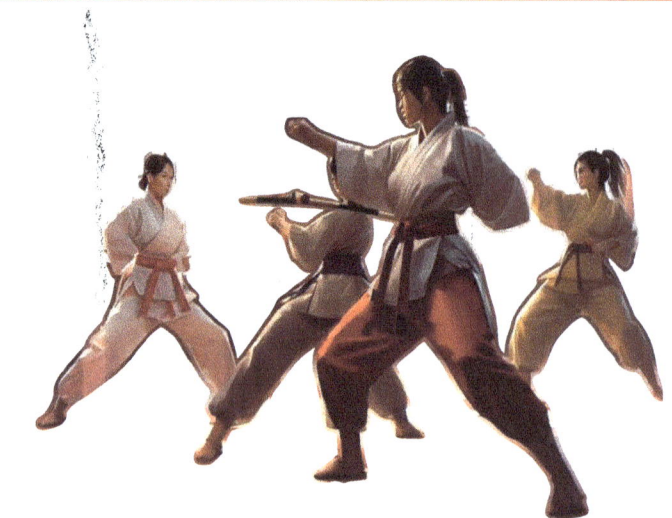

Training in Mixed Martial Arts (MMA) at the Universal Grappling Academy offers numerous benefits specifically for women, addressing various aspects of personal development and empowerment. Here are some reasons why women should consider training in MMA:

1. Safety and Awareness: MMA training enhances situational awareness and teaches practical self-defense techniques, equipping women with the skills to protect themselves in potentially dangerous situations.

2. Self-Confidence: Regular training boosts self-esteem and confidence. As women learn and master new skills, they gain a sense of accomplishment that translates into all areas of life.

3. Domestic Violence Prevention: By learning self-defense techniques, women can feel more empowered and secure in their daily lives, helping to prevent situations of domestic violence and abuse.

4. Self-Defense: MMA teaches effective self-defense strategies that can be used in real-life situations. Understanding how to defend oneself can provide peace of mind and a sense of security.

5. Weight Management: MMA is an intense workout that promotes weight loss and muscle toning. The diverse training routines keep the workouts engaging, making it easier to achieve and maintain fitness goals.

6. Combat Sports Competition: For those interested in competition, grappling tournaments and MMA provides opportunities to participate in various events. Competing can be a thrilling way to challenge oneself and showcase skills.

7. General Fitness: The comprehensive training involved in MMA improves cardiovascular health, strength, flexibility, and overall fitness. It's an excellent way to stay active and healthy while having fun.

Overall, training at the Universal Grappling Academy can be a transformative experience for women, empowering them physically and mentally while building a supportive community.

BEAT THE BULLY

A Guide to Anti-Bullying

It's Better to be Prepared, than to be a Victim

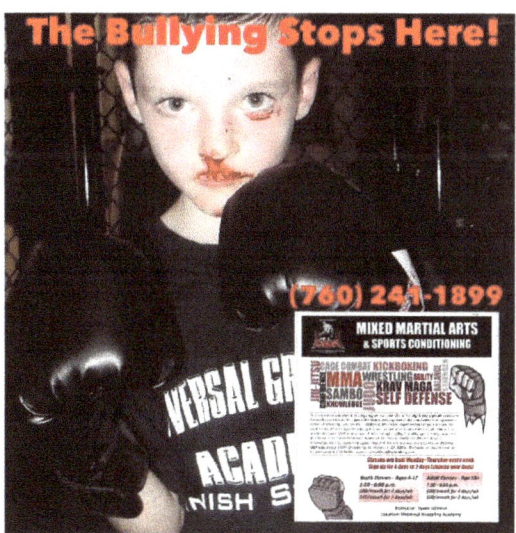

1 – What is a Bully
A bully is typically defined as a person who uses their power, strength, or influence to intimidate, harass, or harm others, often repeatedly. Bullying can take various forms, including physical aggression, verbal abuse, social exclusion, and cyberbullying. The intent behind bullying is usually to establish dominance or control over the victim, leading to emotional and psychological harm. It can occur in various environments, such as schools, workplaces, and online platforms. Addressing bullying involves promoting empathy, communication, and supportive environments to prevent and stop such behavior.

2 – Train for the Bully
Training for a bully can mean preparing yourself to handle bullying situations effectively with intellectual or combat skills learned at the Universal Grappling Academy, whether you are the target of bullying or want to support someone who is. **Regular Exercise:** Engage daily in physical activities like UGA-MMA, which can improve your physical strength and mental resilience.

3 – Build your Confidence
Self-Defense Classes: Consider taking self-defense classes at the Universal Grappling Academy, which can empower you physically and mentally.

Positive Affirmations: Practice positive self-talk to boost your confidence and self-esteem.

4 – Outsmart the Bully
Develop Communication Skills
Assertive Communication: Learn how to express your feelings and needs clearly and confidently without being aggressive.
Role-Playing: Practice responses to bullies with friends or family to prepare for real situations.

Understand the Situation
Recognize Bullying Behaviors: Educate yourself about what constitutes bullying and understand that it's not your fault.
- *Identify Triggers:* Be aware of situations or environments where bullying is more likely to occur.
Practice Conflict Resolution
- *Problem-Solving Skills:* **Learn how to approach conflicts calmly and find solutions that do not involve escalation.**
- *Stay Calm:* Practice techniques for staying calm under pressure, such as deep breathing or counting to ten.

5 – Intimidate the Bully
Focus on Personal Growth
- The bully wants someone who is weak and easily intimidated. If you show strength and confidence, then they are less likely to choose you as their victim.
- *Hobbies and Interests:* **Invest your time in the UGA along with other sports that you enjoy and excel in, which can boost your self-esteem.**
- *Set Personal Goals:* **Work on personal development goals that focus on building strengths, resilience, and combat sports achievements. Posting these achievements will let the bully see that you are a hard worker and an even harder target.**

Training to handle bullying involves a combination of developing physical, intellectual, and personal skills, seeking support, and fostering a positive environment. Remember, it's important to prioritize your safety and well-being above all else.

CHAPTER 9

A FAMILY THAT TRAINS TOGETHER

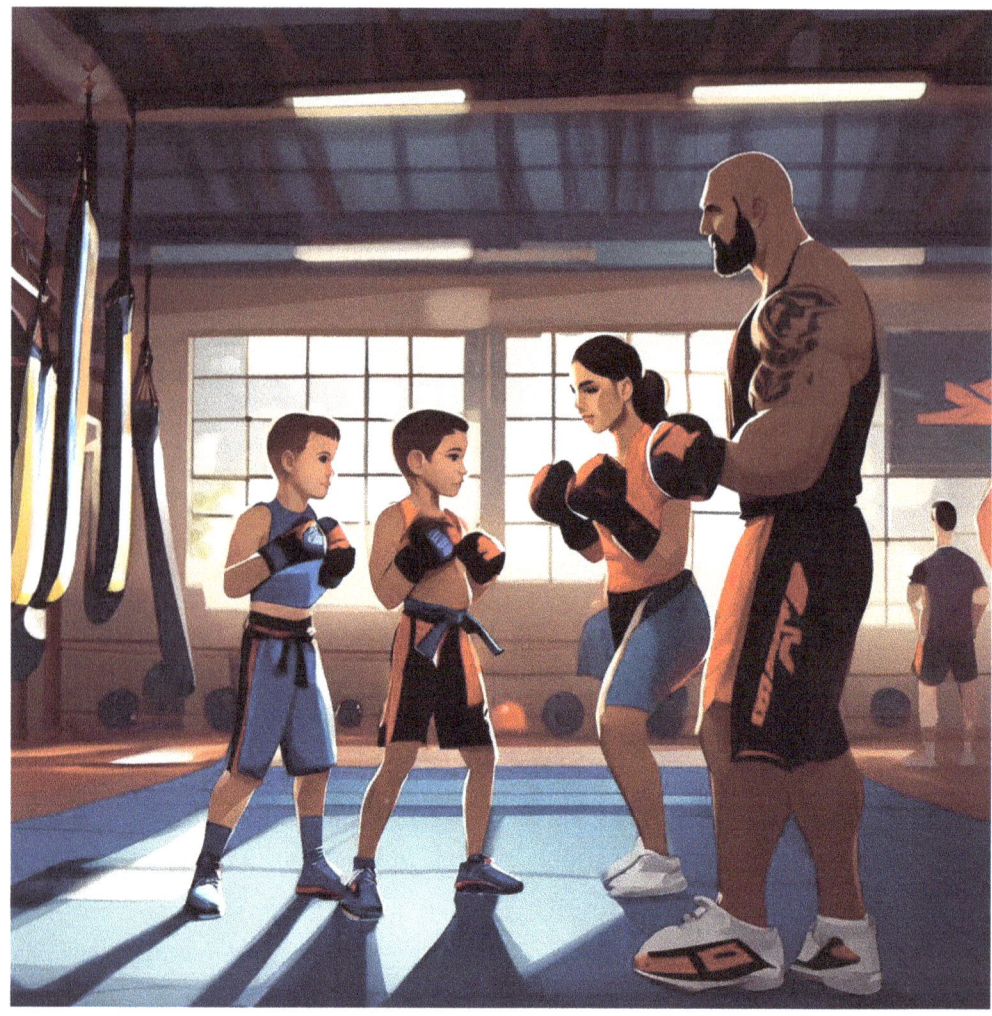

Coach Tyson says: "It's Better to Be Prepared, Rather than to Be A Victim".

I always like to suggest that, if possible, all members of a family should train together. This gives them all the same understanding of what is being taught and allows them to assist each other in their Martial Arts/self-defense growth. I believe and support that Parents should always be involved in their children's learning and competition journey.

Having the entire family train together at the Universal Grappling Academy can be incredibly beneficial for many reasons:

Improved Fitness

1. Shared Physical Activity: Training together encourages a more active lifestyle for the whole family. It promotes fitness in a fun and engaging way, making it easier for everyone to stay motivated.

2. Variety of Skills: Family UGA training sessions can introduce members to various techniques and workouts, fostering a well-rounded approach to fitness & self-defense.

Self-Defense Skills

1. Safety Awareness: Learning self-defense as a family enhances the understanding of personal safety and awareness, equipping everyone with skills to protect themselves in real-life situations.

2. Confidence Building: Training together can boost each family member's confidence, knowing they have the skills to defend themselves and support one another. Hopefully, you'll never need to, but it's better to be prepared than to be a victim.

Family Unity

1. Quality Time: Training together provides a unique opportunity for families to bond. Shared experiences can strengthen relationships and create lasting memories.

2. Teamwork: Grappling and martial arts often emphasize teamwork and support, teaching family members to work together, communicate effectively, and rely on one another.

3. Shared Goals: Setting and achieving fitness and self-defense goals as a family can foster a sense of unity and collective achievement.

Understanding Coach Tyson's Techniques

1. Unified Learning: When families train together, everyone learns the same techniques and philosophies taught by Coach Tyson Johnson. This ensures that all members are on the same page regarding training methods and objectives.

2. Enhanced Communication: Families can discuss and practice techniques learned in class, reinforcing the lessons and improving understanding.

3. Supportive Environment: A family training together creates a supportive learning environment where members can encourage each other, ask questions, and provide constructive feedback.

Overall Development

1. Character Building: Martial arts training often emphasizes discipline, respect, and perseverance. Training as a family allows these values to permeate through family life.

2. Stress Relief: Physical activity is a great way to relieve stress from school, work, or other life experiences. Family training can provide an outlet for expressing emotions and frustrations in a healthy way.

3. Lifelong Skills: The skills learned in UGA grappling extend beyond the mats. The discipline, respect, and confidence gained can positively impact family members 'lives both personally and professionally.

In summary, training together at the Universal Grappling Academy can significantly enhance fitness, self-defense skills, family unity, and understanding of the coaching techniques provided by Coach Tyson Johnson. It creates a holistic experience that benefits every family member both on and off the mats.

Supporting Your Children

Parental support and involvement in their children's training at the Universal Grappling Academy can have a profound impact on the children's overall experience and development. Here are some reasons why it's important for parents to support and possibly train alongside their children:

1. Encouragement and Motivation

- *Boosting Confidence:* When parents actively participate in training, it shows their children that they value the activity, which can enhance the children's confidence and motivation.
- *Positive Reinforcement:* Parents can provide encouragement during and after training sessions, helping children feel supported in their efforts.

2. Shared Experience

- *Bonding Opportunity:* Training together creates shared experiences that can strengthen the parent-child relationship. This time spent together can lead to deeper connections and understanding.
- *Creating Memories:* The shared journey of learning martial arts can create lasting memories that families cherish.

3. Understanding Challenges

- *Empathy for Struggles:* By participating in training, parents can better understand the challenges their children face, fostering empathy and communication about difficulties in learning.
- *Modeling Resilience:* Parents training alongside their children can demonstrate resilience and perseverance, teaching children how to overcome obstacles.

4. Learning Together

- *Unified Learning:* When parents train with their children, they both learn the same techniques and principles, which can enhance discussions about training at home.
- *Supportive Practice:* Parents can help their children practice techniques outside of class, reinforcing what they've learned and improving skills together.

5. Safety and Self-Defense

- *Increased Awareness:* Parents who understand the techniques taught can better discuss safety and self-defense strategies with their children, ensuring they both feel prepared.
- *Joint Self-Defense Skills:* Training together equips both parents and children with essential self-defense skills, fostering confidence in their ability to protect themselves.

6. Creating a Positive Environment

- *Encouraging Active Lifestyles:* When parents engage in physical activities like grappling, they set a positive example for their children, promoting an active and healthy lifestyle.

- *Family Unity:* Shared goals in training can foster a sense of unity and teamwork within the family, enhancing overall family dynamics.

7. Commitment to Growth

- *Demonstrating Commitment:* Parents who participate in their children's martial arts training show their commitment to their children's growth, reinforcing the importance of dedication and hard work.
- *Building Life Skills:* Training in martial arts teaches valuable life skills such as discipline, respect, and focus, which parents can reinforce through their own involvement.

8. Fun and Engagement

- *Enjoyable Activity:* Training together can be a fun and engaging way to spend time as a family, making the experience enjoyable for both parents and children.
- *Healthy Competition:* Sparring or practicing techniques can introduce a playful element of competition, fostering camaraderie and excitement.

In summary, parental support and participation in their children's training at the Universal Grappling Academy can significantly enhance the learning experience. It fosters motivation, understanding, and unity, while also teaching important life skills and creating lasting memories. By being involved, parents not only contribute to their children's growth but also enrich their own lives through shared experiences in martial arts.

Chapter 10
WHITEBOARD KNOWLEDGE

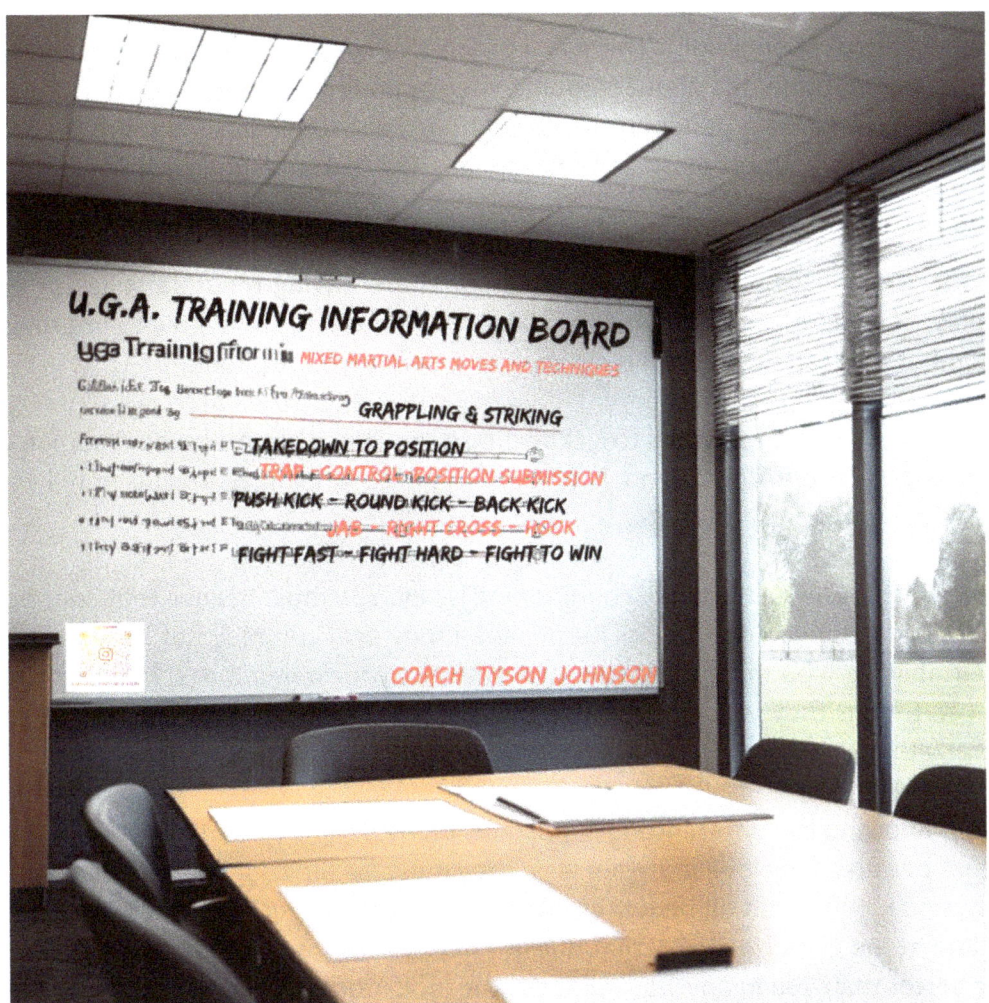

This is where you'll get various information and increase your combat sports IQ / Knowledge from the whiteboard that is hanging in the UGA (Victorville) facility.

Quote: "Don't be Afraid to Compete, be Afraid to Lose"

* From the Coach: If you train hard and focus on everything in this book, you'll have the confidence and the skills to defend yourself, compete, and win almost any engagement that you enter into. If you're afraid to lose, that will hopefully be your motivation to train hard and always do your best at practice and in competition.

Technique - Speed - Power: Develop your technique first; you must know how to do the move properly. After knowing the steps it takes to get to that position or move, you'll work on doing it faster and smoother. Don't power yourself into the move because you'll just end up gassing yourself out. Save your power for the finish and get your submission!

Controlled Aggression: Don't be a Fish...Just flopping around. Every move must have a purpose; don't just do random moves in hopes that they work. Every move must lead to the next position or submission. Make sure that you stay active and moving towards the finish.

Be Persistent: You must constantly be working to get your control position and, of course, the submission. Work for what you want at all times.

T.C.P.S.: Trap, Control, Position, Submission - There is a process of steps to be taken to win in a grappling match or combat sports competition. It's about trapping your opponent's limb(s), be sure to have control to where they cannot easily get away, be sure to have them in the proper position, and then finish your submission. This is all done with your proper technique, speed, and then finished with power.

* Transitions - Improve your method of combat: You may be good at a certain method/style of combat, but be assured that there is always someone better. This is where having multiple styles or methods of combat comes into play…If someone is better at something, you'll need to know how to improvise and use a different style of combat that can (hopefully) overcome and defeat your opponent.

For Example: if they have better boxing, switch to kickboxing; if they have better kickboxing than you switch to wrestling or judo to take them down, and if they're good at wrestling, maybe you'll have better submission skills from the ground positions, etc.

Outwork Your Opponent: This is where optimal conditioning is key. You must believe that your opponent(s) are working their asses off and if you don't work harder then they are, you may not be able to drain their conditioning and their abilities. You must out-move and outwork your opponent(s) in order to push their conditioning. If you can't, then they will gain the upper hand when you've fatigued, even if you are the better grappler/fighter/athlete.

Shape vs Conditioning: Knowing the difference is important, many people get intimidated by the shape of a person, believing that because they look a certain way, they must be superior somehow. Shape is just the look of a person's physique, which can all be just smoke and mirrors because of genetics, or yes, because they spend a lot of time at the gym. However, that doesn't necessarily make them good at combat sports, tougher than you, or better than you in any way. Shape is the look, Conditioning is the heart and lungs of a person's physique, and the hard work towards endurance and constant movement. It's the conditioning that'll win the fight and not the shape…I've seen many non-physical specimens destroy the in-shape muscular guys and gals in fights. Looking good doesn't win fights; technique, persistence, and conditioning does.

Opportunity - See it or Create it: You must know how to see when your opponent gives you the opportunity to better your position or a submission. If not, then you'll need to know how to create these opportunities…One great way is to use "Pain Points" or move in certain directions/positions.

Pain Points: These are any points on your opponent's body that do one or more of these things: 1. Create Pain 2. Disrupts your opponent's Thought Process 3. It forces them to make a move (that'll help you better your position or get your submission).

Disruption Before Defense: If you disrupt it, you won't have to defend it. This means that if you know and understand the steps/positions it takes for an opponent to get you into a submission, then you won't have to fight your way out of a submission. Disruption = No Defense because disruption is your Pre-Defense. If you're in a submission move, then that means it's too late, you should have tucked in, taken away their position, their angle, or their hold before they got it locked in.

3 Points of Balance: Head, Shoulders, and Hips - control one, two, or all three of them, and you'll have control of your opponent's body whether you're standing or on the ground. Where the head goes, the body goes; where the shoulders go, the body goes, and where the hips go, the body goes.

Balance and Positioning: Be sure to keep good balance and positioning, whether you're standing or on the ground. Remember, don't cross your feet or stand too wide, keep a good base at all times, along with positions that won't get you rolled or reversed.

* Get it First, Get it Fast, Get it Hard: When in combat, it's important to make the moves first, don't wait for your opponent to strike, they may only need that one move. Be fast, if you don't move faster than they can react or defend, then you need to be faster...Third is to make the first and fast move a hard move...Knock them out/down and make your first move the only move needed in the fight.

Fight to be First: Don't wait to defend, stay active, persistent, and aggressive so you can make all the moves first, which will keep your opponent on the defense.

Body Mechanics: Know the human body, study how the body moves, and how it shouldn't move as well. This will give you more opportunities to find uncommon submissions against your opponent.

Reaction vs Response: A reaction is a defensive move...Your opponent shoots in or throws a punch, and so you'll react with a sprawl or a block...Your response is an offensive move that comes after the reaction. This is where, after you sprawl, you'll get a front choke or spin and take back control, etc. Or after the striking block, you throw some punches/strikes of your own.

Fight or Fear: Getting hit will do one of two things, some call it the " fight or flight" response. So what I am saying is the same difference. When getting hit, people have one of these two reactions. As a fighter, you train daily and are constantly getting hit; this helps you develop the proper response to getting hit, and that would be to fight!

* 3 Zones: Know your zones and what body tools/strikes to use against your opponent(s) zone areas. Zone one is from their feet to their hips. This takes away their power, balance, speed and movement. Zone two is from the hips to the shoulders. This takes away their abilities to breathe, their punching power, and their grappling/striking tools. Zone three is the head and face. Here you'll disrupt their sight, breathing, and possibly their consciousness.

A UGA Fighter should be conditioned, fast, and aggressive: Each fighter should be committed to their goals. Training should be consistent and intense, focusing on strong conditioning for endurance, speed, and a strong desire to win.

Champions Train to be Champions: If you hope to be a champion, you must train to be one. Your Goals don't care about your excuses, so show up, work hard, and be the best that you can be in practice and in combat. Do the work that others aren't willing to do and push yourself to uncomfortable limits. I like to think that, as hard as I am working, my opponent may be working harder, which gives me the motivation to push through even more.

IF Coach is Nagging = Coach is Caring: Listen, I am only on you because I want you to succeed and achieve your goals. My job is to guide you to personal victory and coach you in the various ways to achieve those goals. But, not all people have the same drive, or sometimes they begin to slow down, and that's where a coach is there to nag you a little bit to push you through… If I didn't care, then I wouldn't say anything, and you'd soon give up on yourself when the going got tough.

Basics to Work on: Takedowns, Positive Control Positions (Full Mount - Side Mount - Back Control), Stay out of the Guard, Passing the Guard, Chokes, Arm-Bars, Leg Locks, Wrist Locks, Pain Points, Reversals, Wrist Control, Bulgarian Series, NEVER QUIT…

Stay Cool, Calm, and in Control: When in training or in competition, you must stay in mental control at all times. When a match gets tough and you and your opponent are equally matched, staying calm and keeping a clear head is paramount. When you allow yourself to get frustrated, you cloud your mind up, and it's harder for you to see the clear paths to victory. If you're in quicksand, you can either sink or pull yourself out; a cool and calm head will keep you in control.

Out Move, Out Maneuver, and Out Position Your Opponent: A stiff and still body will never win your combat competition. You must develop superb conditioning so that you can out-move and out-work your opponent using all the techniques that you've learned in practice. This helps to confuse and tire out your opposition while putting the test to their endurance and conditioning.

CHAPTER 11

THE COACHES OFFICE

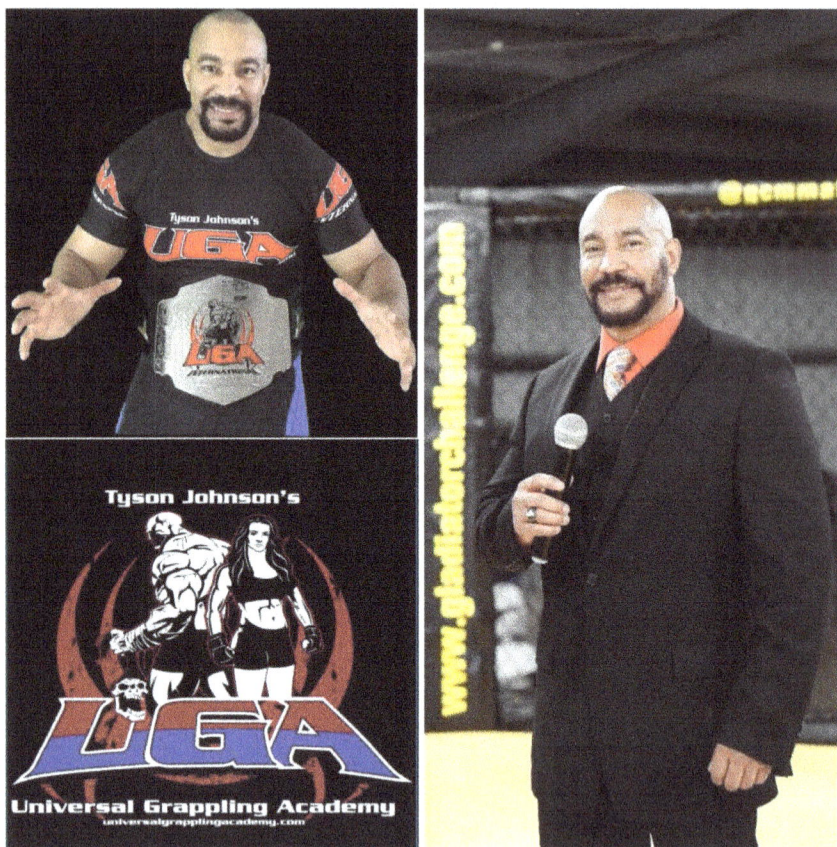

I was told once by another coach, "Don't be friends with your students." To a certain extent, that might be true, but I always try to develop relationships with my students. Obviously, there has to be a dividing line between friendship and business, and I just have to be sure not to cross it.

Being a good coach involves a combination of skills, qualities, and practices that foster a positive and productive environment for athletes or team members. Here are some things that I believe will help as a coach.

1. Communication: Clear and open communication is essential. A good coach should be able to convey instructions, feedback, and encouragement effectively. I talk to my students because I care. A fun, upbeat atmosphere helps keep everyone happy and learning, and sometimes a stern talk can correct behavior.

2. Empathy: Understanding the feelings and perspectives of students/athletes helps build trust and rapport. A coach should be able to relate to their experiences and challenges. Everyone is going through things in life; I try to be understanding as much as I can.

3. Knowledge of the Sport: A solid understanding of the technical aspects of the sport is critical. This includes strategies, rules, and skills necessary for success. A good coach is always a student. I continue to learn and never think that I know enough or everything.

4. Motivation: Inspiring and motivating athletes to perform at their best is a core responsibility. This can be achieved through positive reinforcement, goal setting, and instilling a strong work ethic. That's the UGA way.

5. Adaptability: Every student/athlete is different, and a good coach should be flexible in their approach, tailoring their coaching style to meet individual learning needs and circumstances.

6. Leadership: A good coach leads by example, demonstrating commitment, integrity, and professionalism. They should be able to guide the team both on and off the field. A good coach brings people together for both physical training and personal growth.

7. Patience: Developing skills and building a team takes time. Patience is key when working through challenges and helping athletes progress. Working with children is as challenging as it gets. So many personalities, along with the lack of focus and sometimes interest, will require an amazing amount of patience.

8. Constructive Feedback: Providing feedback that is specific, actionable, and supportive helps athletes improve without discouraging them. Know how to be open-minded and talk to the different personalities that you'll come across.

9. Encouraging Teamwork: Fostering a sense of camaraderie and collaboration among team members enhances performance and creates a positive environment. We are a team and in some ways like family, work hard, motivate, stay loyal, help encourage, and build that team/family.

10. Continuous Learning: A good coach is always looking to improve their coaching skills and knowledge, staying updated with the latest training techniques and trends.

11. Protect the Children: From the Dangers of this world because they are our future, our legacy, and the testament of our commitment to helping children. We help them grow physically, mentally, emotionally, and socially. We teach them how to deal with hard situations and how to have the confidence and courage to defend themselves or others. If we protect them from predators, they'll grow to protect themselves and others from predators. Show them that in life, you can be smart, kind, and patient, but have a switch that can be turned on to handle business when necessary. Teach them how to overcome challenges, setbacks, and rough/tough Competition.

12. Be Understanding: Know and understand that everyone learns differently and/or at a different pace. When working with children, you have to understand that their brains are still developing. Some kids mature faster than others, and at that age, they have so much energy and distractions that you'll need to be patient. Yes, it's difficult sometimes, but try to make the move you're trying to teach them into a fun game or find other ways to teach them. Being understanding and patient will help both you and the children have a better learning experience.

13. Fight the UGA Way: Teach the Students - Don't Fight Afraid, Don't Fight to Survive, Fight to Win. Fight Fast, Hard, and with Accuracy.. Open up and use all of the skills that you've learned to win.

By embodying these qualities and practices, a coach can effectively support their athletes and foster a successful team.

14. A List of things I ask of my Students:

Never Quit - This only leads to failure, not only in your combat sports journey, but in many other things in life that need your dedication and no-quit attitude.

Get comfortable with being uncomfortable - We'll help you push yourself beyond your limits in order to advance your limits. It's not easy, and that's what'll make you different than ordinary people and better than your opponents.

Be Coachable/Teachable/Open to Learning - If you're stubborn, hard-headed, and or A know-it-all, then it'll be difficult to assist you in improving or adding to your skills. Listen, observe, practice, and learn…We're here to help you and guide you towards your personal best, so don't push back from constructive criticism or training methods. You'll only be hurting yourself!

Be a Good Teammate - If you're difficult to work with because of a negative attitude or being too stiff of a partner or unwilling to do things as instructed, then it'll be hard for you to find people or a facility to work with. Stay open, teachable, and helpful to your teammates; we're all on the same team with similar goals that we can all reach together if we work as a unit.

Be a Good Student - You're here to learn and or improve. Respect and Honor your coach, don't steal from or betray your coach in any way, don't talk shit, gossip or develop clicks against the coach or anybody in the facility, this only distracts from everyone's goals and disrupts the positive energy of the facility. If you're unhappy and or not getting what you're looking for, keep it to yourself, cancel properly, and move on to a facility that better suits your needs with dignity and respect.

Challenge Your Limits, You Can't Finish What You Haven't Started - If you are not willing to go above and beyond your current limits in training, how do you expect to beat the opponents that are? If you don't start your journey, how do you ever expect to reach your goals/finish line? "The Best Way to Get Through it, Is to Get To It."

Train the Pain - When you want to stop, you must force yourself to keep going. That's building mental strength! Yes, it hurts, it sucks, but if you quit, then you'll never make it, if you go farther, then every little step is a step of progress. Pain is your friend/weakness leaving the body, and any ordinary person can quit on themselves. You're training to be an extraordinary athlete.

Believe in Yourself - This is half the battle. Self-belief, which means that you can overcome the many battles in practice and in competition, will help you get through life. It won't get easier; you'll just get stronger, so remember that your goals were meant to be broken and will only be broken if you believe that you can push through the hard times.

You Create Your Future - If you want it, you can get it, but it'll take hard work, Desire, Determination, and Dedication. The work you put in today will lay the path to your future. Greatness comes to those who work towards it.

15. Trust the Process
- Success won't come overnight. It takes time, work, and dedication to play the long game in order for your success to show. Trust that your coach knows what he's doing and that his methods are designed to help you achieve your goals. You need to stay focused, determined, and hard at work in order to progress and see the fruits of your labor. If you stay on a path, it'll get you where you want to go,

but if you get distracted or try to take shortcuts, then your progress could come much slower.. Be Patient and Trust the Process.

16. 100% Capacity - When training in Combat Sports, it is almost impossible to be at 100% all the time and without soreness or injury. What I say is that you may not be at 100%, but just give 100% of whatever you have every time you train.

17. Losing is Learning - Nobody likes to lose, I hate losing, but in order to improve your chance of NOT losing, you must use those unfortunate situations to learn. You must learn and outsmart your opponent as well as avoid the loss. Figure it out…How did you lose? What steps did your opponent take in order to defeat you? What steps can you take to prevent it from happening again? Was it your conditioning, was your opponent just better than you(faster, stronger, more technical), was it just a slip-up or something that you missed in practice? Figure it out and overcome that obstacle so that it doesn't happen again. So if a loss occurs, be determined not to repeat it, stay mentally strong, study it, and improve on whatever your weakness in that area was..

18. A good coach is always a student - If a coach believes that he/she is the best in the world, knows everything, resists alternative or modern techniques or training methods, then it's possible that you have the wrong coach. A good coach should have your best interests in mind and must always be open to adaptation. Not all students learn in the same way or there may be alternate ways to improve a skill or move; in this case, the coach should learn the benefits of a new method and find the best way to incorporate it into their training. As a coach, "if you're done learning and growing, you'll soon find yourself and program slowing" 😃 A coach should stay up to date on new techniques and training options to keep themselves and their program relevant.

19. Children are Sponges - Like a sponge, that soaks up water, a child's mind is the same. Help make sure that everything that they soak up in their young, growing minds is positive and constructive for their future. Hard work, respect, loyalty, responsibility, confidence, knowledge, etc. Help them to grow up properly and to be productive members of society. Children soak up what they see and hear as they grow, which means that their behavior is fueled by the lifestyle that they grow up with at home. Fuel them with a healthy lifestyle, good hearts, and minds.

20. Procrastination - If you're not moving forward, you'll never arrive at your location or achieve your goals. Your goals don't care about your excuses, so if you sit in quicksand, you'll stay where you are. Pull yourself up and out, move forward with what you want in life. Even little steps forward are progress, so find your way forward and don't let your excuses take your time away; you need to progress.

21. Embrace the Challenge - When attempting to achieve a goal, your biggest obstacle is going to be you. You must be mentally strong and convince yourself that the goal is obtainable. You must believe in yourself, work hard, and never accept defeat. Embrace the challenge that's ahead of you, go after it, and have a fantastic time overcoming the struggles and defeating that challenge until you reach your goal.

22. Don't Quit - I don't care how tough it is, you'll never lose if you don't quit! Work hard through thick and thin. If you get defeated in a match, come back and work harder. No matter what you go through in competition or in life, you'll never be a loser unless you quit.

23. Age is Just a Number - We've trained people of all ages and assisted them in reaching their goals. Two men were in their upper 50s, and both had aspirations to fight in the cage. Both of them came to the UGA, trained hard, and achieved their goals; they both competed in MMA fights. Don't say you can't do something unless you just don't want to try. Age is no excuse for you to fail; set your goals and go after them.

24. Discipline at a Young Age - Teach them at a young age that there are consequences for their actions, both good and bad. If you enable a child to act disrespectfully at home, they'll be disrespectful in public. Let them know that you are in charge and they must do as you say without attitude or backtalk. A disrespectful child will grow to be a disrespectful teen/adult. If you can't handle them now, how will you handle them when they're much older, bigger, and stronger?

Life can either be easy or hard, and that depends on the choices they make. Show them that making the proper choices will result in good responses, but making bad choices will result in negative responses. It's like making the difference between grappling on the mat (good choices) or grappling on the pavement (bad choices). Get them used to honoring and being respectful to their parents, teachers, law enforcement, etc., so that their journey in life will be made with good choices and much easier outcomes.

By embodying these qualities and practices, a coach and the students can effectively support their program/lives and foster a successful team.

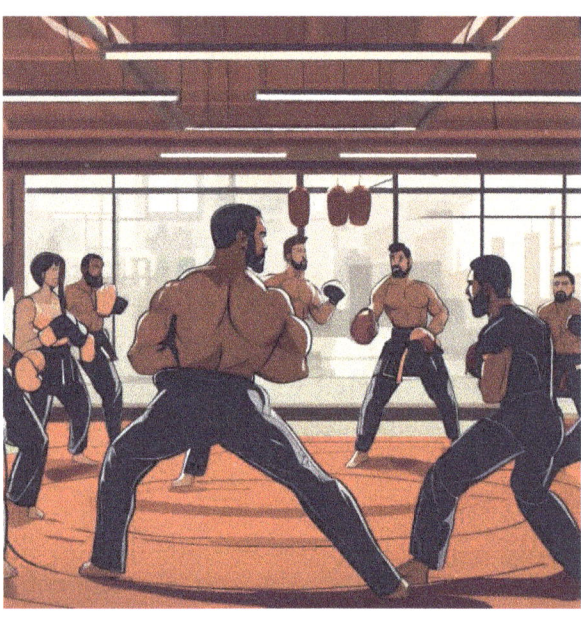

CHAPTER 12
UGA TRAINING ROUTINES

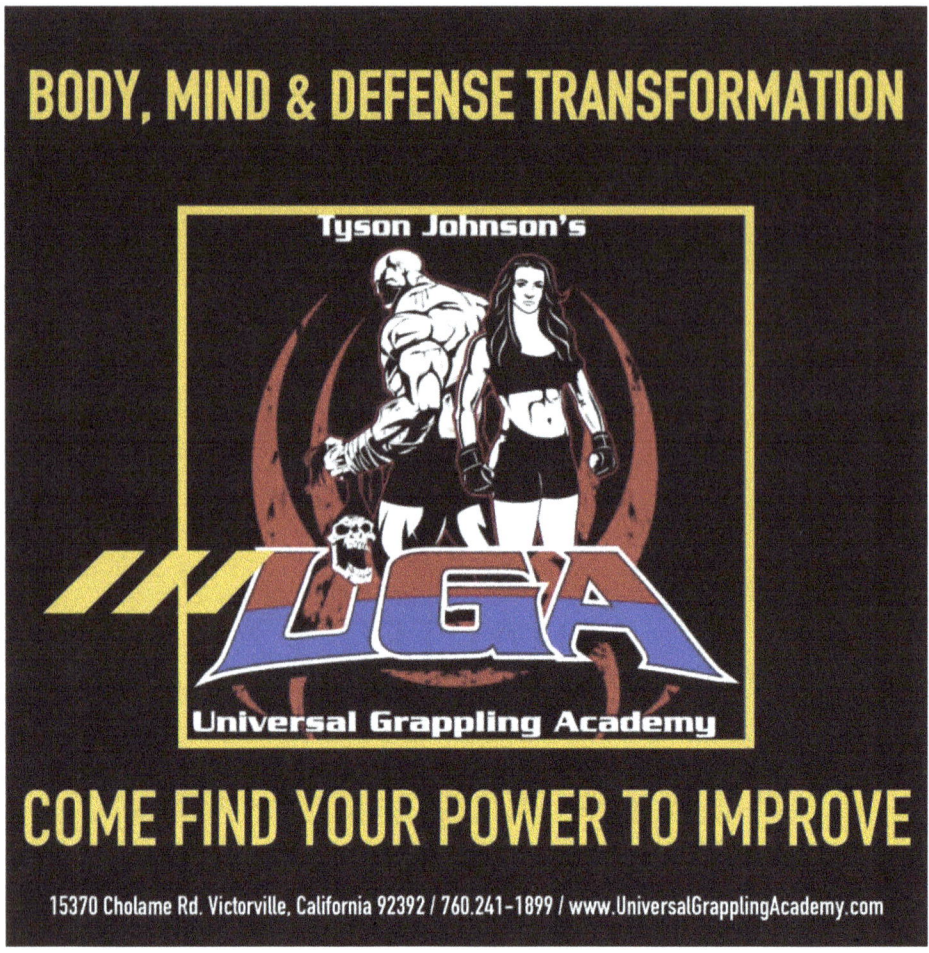

Embark on a transformative journey with "The UGA Athlete's Training Guide," where coach Tyson Johnson reveals a treasure trove of authentic workout and nutrition routines designed specifically for the Universal Grappling Academy.

This essential guide is tailored for both novice and experienced athletes in combat sports, but its principles extend far beyond the mat, benefitting anyone striving for excellence in their sport and personal life.

In this comprehensive guide, you will find a diverse array of proven training programs and nutritional strategies that have been meticulously crafted to empower ordinary individuals to become extraordinary athletes. Tyson Johnson's innovative approach emphasizes the importance of consistent practice, effective recovery, and a champion's mindset, providing you with the tools needed to unlock your full potential.

Whether your goal is to enhance your grappling skills, improve your overall fitness, or cultivate the resilience needed to face life's challenges, "The UGA Athlete's Training Guide" is your ultimate resource. Discover how these remarkable programs can lead you to peak performance and personal success, turningyour aspirations into reality. Step into the realm of greatness and let the UGA philosophy inspire your journey!

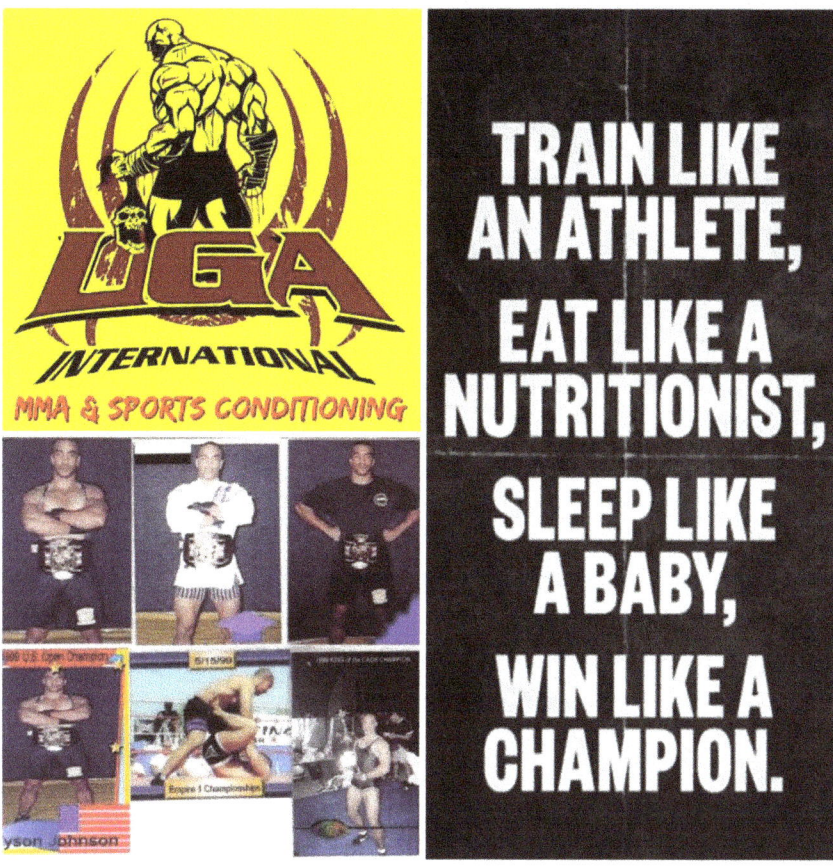

UGA GRAPPLING TOURNAMENT PREPARATION

1. Training Regimen:
   - *Technique Drilling:* Focus on specific techniques and moves. Practice all the drills on the opposite side of this page. Practice your favorite submissions, escapes, and takedowns.
   - *Sparring:* Engage in live sparring sessions as much as possible with someone as good or better than you to apply techniques under pressure. Change your partners to experience different styles.
   - *Conditioning:* Incorporate strength and conditioning workouts to improve endurance, strength, and agility. Focus on exercises that mimic grappling movements.

2. Nutrition:
   - *Balanced Diet:* Eat a balanced diet rich in proteins, carbohydrates, and healthy fats. Incorporate plenty of fruits and vegetables.
   - *Hydration:* Stay well-hydrated in the days leading up to the tournament. Proper hydration improves performance and recovery.
   - *Weight Management:* If you're competing in a weight class, monitor your weight and adjust your diet accordingly.

3. Mental Preparation:
   - *Visualization:* Spend time visualizing your matches, including executing techniques and overcoming challenges.

- *Mindfulness:* Practice mindfulness or meditation to help manage anxiety and improve focus.

4. Tactical Planning:
   - *Analyze Opponents:* If possible, watch the styles of potential opponents. Look for their strengths and weaknesses.
   - *Game Plan:* Develop a game plan for your matches, including your preferred moves and adjustments you might need to make.

5. Gear and Equipment:
   - *Check Your Gear:* Ensure you have all necessary gear, such as your UGA shorts, UGA rash guard, mouthguard, and any protective gear. Make sure everything fits well.
   - *Competition Rules:* Familiarize yourself with the tournament rules and regulations, including scoring and illegal moves.

6. Recovery:
   - *Rest:* Prioritize rest and recovery in the days leading up to the tournament. Avoid heavy training the day before, just work conditioning and techniques.
   - *Stretching and Mobility:* Incorporate stretching and mobility work to keep your body limber and reduce the risk of injury. Flexibility is important in grappling.

7. Day of the Tournament:
   - *Plan Your Day:* Arrive early to the venue, allowing time for warm-up and mental preparation.
   - *Stay Calm:* Focus on your breathing and stay relaxed. Trust your coach, training, and enjoy the experience of testing your skills and getting that Gold Medal, Sword, or Belt….

By following these steps, you can increase your chances of success in the tournament. Stay UGA Strong…..Good luck!

UNIVERSAL GRAPPLING ACADEMY

Cardio and Conditioning Routine

Warm-Up (5-10 minutes)
- Jog in place or brisk walking
- Arm circles (30 seconds forward and 30 seconds backward)
- Leg swings (30 seconds each leg)
- Dynamic stretches (lunges, torso twists)

Circuit Workout (Repeat 3-4 times)

1. Jumping Jacks (90 seconds)
  - Boosts heart rate and warms up the body.

2. Push-Ups (30 seconds)
  - Works on upper body strength. Modify by doing them on your knees if necessary.

3. High Knees (90 seconds)
  - Stand in place and run while bringing your knees up to waist level.

4. Bodyweight Squats (90 seconds)
  - Focus on proper form to engage the lower body.

5. Burpees (30 seconds)
  - A full-body exercise that combines a squat, push-up, and jump.

6. Plank (1 minute)
  - Strengthens the core. Hold a traditional plank or modify on your knees.

7. Mountain Climbers (1 minute)
  - Get into a push-up position and alternate bringing your knees to your chest.

8. Lateral Shuffles (1 minute)
  - Shuffle side to side quickly to improve agility.

Cool Down (5-10 minutes)
- Slow walking to bring the heart rate down
- Stretching major muscle groups (hold each stretch for 15-30 seconds)
  - Hamstring stretch
  - Quadriceps stretch
  - Shoulder stretch
  - Triceps stretch

Tips:
- Stay hydrated throughout the routine.
- Listen to your body; modify exercises as needed.
- Gradually increase the intensity and duration as your fitness improves.
- Aim for at least 3-4 sessions per week for optimal results.

UGA - PowerLifting Routine

Here's a 5-day PowerLifting routine that focuses on the three lifts: Squats, Bench Press, and Deadlifts, while incorporating accessory work to build overall strength and support muscle growth.

Day 1: Squat Focus
- *Back Squat:* 4 sets of 6 reps
- *Front Squat:* 3 sets of 6 reps
- *Leg Press:* 3 sets of 8-10 reps
- *Romanian Deadlifts:* 3 sets of 8 reps
- *Calf Raises:* 4 sets of 12-15 reps
- *Core Work:* Planks, 3 sets for 30-60 seconds

Day 2: Bench Press Focus
- *Bench Press:* 4 sets of 6 reps
- *Incline Dumbbell Press:* 3 sets of 8 reps
- *Dumbbell Flyes:* 3 sets of 10-12 reps
- *Tricep Dips:* 3 sets of 8-10 reps
- *Face Pulls:* 3 sets of 12-15 reps
- *Core Work:* Hanging Leg Raises, 3 sets of 10-15 reps

Day 3: Deadlift Focus
- *Deadlift:* 4 sets of 6 reps
- *Deficit Deadlifts:* 3 sets of 5 reps
- *Barbell Rows:* 3 sets of 6-8 reps
- *Pull-Ups or Lat Pulldowns:* 3 sets of 8-10 reps
- *Hyperextensions:* 3 sets of 10-12 reps
- *Core Work:* Russian Twists, 3 sets of 10-15 reps per side

Day 4: Volume and Accessory Work
- *Squat (light):* 3 sets of 8-10 reps
- *Bench Press (light):* 3 sets of 8-10 reps
- *Leg Curls:* 3 sets of 10-12 reps
- *Lateral Raises:* 3 sets of 12-15 reps
- *Bicep Curls:* 3 sets of 10-12 reps
- *Core Work:* Ab Wheel Rollouts, 3 sets of 8-10 reps

Day 5: Combined Technique and Conditioning
- *Pause Squats:* 3 sets of 5 reps
- *Close Grip Bench Press:* 3 sets of 6-8 reps
- *Sumo Deadlifts:* 3 sets of 5 reps
- *Battle Ropes or Conditioning Circuits:* 10-15 minutes
- *Mobility Work:* 15-20 minutes of stretching and foam rolling

Notes:
- Ensure proper warm-up before each session (dynamic stretching, light cardio).
- Focus on technique, especially for the main lifts.
- Adjust weights according to your personal level and progress.
- Rest 1-2 minutes between sets for main lifts and 30-60 seconds for accessory work.
- Include a rest day or active recovery day as needed.

UGA - MMA Beginning Class

A beginner's mixed martial arts (MMA) training course involves designing a structured program that covers fundamental techniques, conditioning, and practical application. Here`s a 10-week course:

Course Overview
Duration: 10 weeks
Frequency: 2 classes per week (1.5 hours each)
Target Audience: Beginners with no prior experience

* *Week 1: Introduction to MMA*
- *Class 1:* Orientation
  - *Overview of MMA:* History, rules, and disciplines (striking, grappling)
  - Importance of safety and respect in training
  - Basic warm-up and stretching routines

- * *Class 2: Stance and Movement*
  - Basic fighting stances (orthodox and southpaw)
  - Footwork fundamentals (advancing, retreating, lateral movement)
  - Basic shadowboxing drills

* *Week 2: Striking Basics*
- *Class 3:* Boxing Fundamentals
  - Introduction to punches (jab, cross, hook, uppercut)
  - Basic combinations and defensive movements (slipping, bobbing, weaving)

- *Class 4: Kicking Techniques*
  - Basic kicks (front kick, roundhouse kick, side kick)

- How to deliver and retract kicks safely
- Kicking drills and pad work

Week 3: Grappling Fundamentals
- **Class 5:** Introduction to Grappling
  - Basic positions (guard, mount, side control)
  - Introduction to takedowns (single leg, double leg)

- **Class 6: Escapes and Submissions**
  - Escaping from common positions (guard, mount)
  - Introduction to basic submissions (arm-bar, rear-naked choke)

Week 4: Combining Techniques
- **Class 7:** Striking and Movement
  - Integrating footwork with striking
  - Partner drills for combinations

- **Class 8: Takedowns and Transitions**
  - Practicing takedowns in combination with strikes
  - Drilling transitions between striking and grappling

Week 5: Basic Sparring and Conditioning
- **Class 9:** Controlled Sparring
  - Introduction to light sparring with partners
  - Emphasis on technique over power

- **Class 10: Conditioning and Strength Training**
  - MMA-specific conditioning drills (interval training, agility drills)
  - Bodyweight strength exercises (push-ups, squats, planks)

Week 6: Advanced Striking Techniques
- **Class 11:** Elbows and Knees
  - Introduction to elbow strikes and knee strikes
  - Drills to practice these techniques in different ranges

- **Class 12: Defense in Striking**
  - Defensive techniques (blocking, parrying, countering)
  - Partner drills for defensive movements

Week 7: Advanced Grappling Techniques
- **Class 13:** Takedown Defense
  - Techniques for defending against takedowns
  - Drills for maintaining balance and positioning

- *Class 14: Advanced Submissions*
  - Introduction to more complex submissions (triangle choke, guillotine)
  - Partner drills for applying submissions

Week 8: Strategy and Fight Simulation
- *Class 15:* Fight Strategy Basics
  - Discussing fight strategy and fight IQ
  - Analyzing fights and techniques

- *Class 16: Sparring Practice*
  - Structured sparring sessions with feedback
  - Emphasis on applying learned techniques in a controlled environment

Week 9: Review and Skill Refinement
- *Class 17:* Technique Review
  - Review of all techniques learned in previous weeks
  - Focus on correcting mistakes and refining skills

- *Class 18: Conditioning and Sparring*
  - High-intensity conditioning drills
  - Sparring with a focus on applying techniques under fatigue

Week 10: Graduation and Future Steps
- *Class 19:* Showcase Sparring
  - Participants showcase their skills in a friendly sparring session
  - Feedback from instructors and peers

- *Class 20: Course Wrap-Up*
  - Discussion on progression in MMA (next steps, advanced classes)
  - Graduation ceremony and certificates

Additional Components
- *Supplemental Materials:* Handouts on techniques, nutrition, and fitness tips.
- *Safety Gear:* Ensure all participants have proper gear (gloves, shin guards, mouth guard).
- *Instructor Availability:* Encourage participants to ask questions and seek feedback.

This beginner's MMA course structure provides a comprehensive introduction to the sport while ensuring safety and skill development.

UGA Intermediate Training Program

Here's an intermediate mixed martial arts training program designed to enhance your skills, strength, and conditioning. This program includes a mix of striking, grappling, and conditioning workouts, along with rest days for recovery.

Weekly Training Schedule

Monday: Striking Focus
- *Warm-up (15 min):* Jump rope, dynamic stretches.
- *Technique (30 min):*
  - *Shadowboxing (5 rounds, 3 min each)*
  - *Heavy bag work (5 rounds, 3 min each)*
  - *Focus mitt drills with a partner (4 rounds, 2 min each)*
- *Conditioning (15 min):*
  - *HIIT (High-Intensity Interval Training):* 20 sec work, 10 sec rest, 8 rounds (burpees, mountain climbers, and squat jumps).

Tuesday: Grappling Focus
- *Warm-up (15 min):* Movement drills, partner stretching.
- *Technique (30 min):*
  - *Drilling takedowns* (single/double leg) and defenses (5 rounds, 5 min each).
  - *Positional sparring* (5 rounds, 3 min each, focusing on guard and mount positions).
- *Conditioning (15 min):*
  - *Circuit training* (push-ups, pull-ups, kettlebell swings, and lunges).

Wednesday: Rest and Recovery
- *Active recovery:* Light jogging or yoga for flexibility.

Thursday: Mixed Techniques
- *Warm-up (15 min):* Agility drills.
- *Technique (30 min):*
  - *Combination drills* (striking into takedown).
  - *Sparring* (3 rounds, 5 min each, alternating roles with a partner).
- *Conditioning (15 min):*
  - *Plyometric exercises* (box jumps, plyo push-ups, jump squats).

Friday: Sparring and Strategy
- *Warm-up (15 min):* Jump rope and mobility exercises.
- *Sparring (45 min):*
  - Round-robin sparring with various partners (3 rounds, 5 min each).
  - Focus on applying techniques learned throughout the week.
- *Cool down (15 min):* Stretching and foam rolling.

Saturday: Strength and Conditioning
- *Warm-up (10 min):* Dynamic stretches.
- *Strength Training (30 min):*
  - *Compound lifts* (deadlifts, squats, bench press).
  - *Core exercises* (planks, Russian twists, medicine ball throws).
- *Cardio (20 min):*
  - *Steady-state cardio* (running, cycling).

Sunday: Rest and Mental Training
- *Focus on mental preparation:* Visualization, meditation, or reviewing fight footage.

* Additional Tips
- *Hydration and Nutrition:* Maintain a balanced diet rich in protein, carbohydrates, and healthy fats. Stay hydrated.
- *Listen to Your Body:* Adjust the intensity and volume based on your recovery and energy levels.
- *Supplementary Skills:* Consider adding yoga or Pilates for flexibility and core strength.

Feel free to modify this program based on your specific goals or available resources!

UGA - Advanced MMA Training Course

Here's an advanced mixed martial arts training course designed to push your skills, conditioning, and tactical understanding to the next level. This program includes specialized training in striking, grappling, and advanced conditioning, along with recovery and mental training components.

Advanced MMA Training Course Outline

Duration: 8 Weeks
Frequency: 5 Training Days per Week

Weekly Training Schedule

Monday: Advanced Striking Techniques
- *Warm-up (15 min):* Agility drills, shadowboxing.
- *Technique (30 min):*
  - *Advanced combinations* (4 rounds, 3 min each) incorporating angles and footwork.
  - *Partner drills on counters and feints* (4 rounds, 2 min each).
- *Sparring (30 min):*
  - Controlled sparring focusing on implementing new techniques (4 rounds, 5 min each).
- *Conditioning (15 min):*
  - *HIIT:* 30 sec work, 15 sec rest, 6 rounds (focus on explosive movements).

Tuesday: Advanced Grappling and Takedowns
- *Warm-up (15 min):* Movement drills, partner stretching.
- *Technique (30 min):*
  - Takedown variations and counters (5 rounds, 5 min each).
  - Guard passing drills with resistance (4 rounds, 3 min each).
- *Live Sparring (30 min):*
  - Focus on positional sparring from various positions (4 rounds, 5 min each).
- *Conditioning (15 min):*
  - Circuit training (battle ropes, kettlebell swings, and agility ladder drills).

Wednesday: Tactical Sparring and Strategy
- *Warm-up (15 min):* Dynamic stretches and footwork drills.
- *Sparring (60 min):*
  - Structured sparring sessions with specific goals (e.g., focusing on defense, takedowns, or submissions).
- *Cooldown and Analysis (15 min):* Review sparring footage or partner feedback.

Thursday: Mixed Techniques and Strategy
- *Warm-up (15 min):* Jump rope and mobility exercises.
- *Technique (30 min):*
  - Integrating striking into grappling (5 rounds, 5 min each).
  - Scramble drills to improve transitions (4 rounds, 3 min each).
- *Conditioning (30 min):*
  - Strength training focused on explosive lifts (clean and press, snatch).
  - Core conditioning (medicine ball slams, hanging leg raises).

Friday: Fight Simulation and Conditioning
- *Warm-up (15 min):* Light jogging followed by dynamic stretches.
- *Fight Simulation (60 min):*
  - Sparring sessions mimicking fight conditions (3-5 rounds, 5 min each with 1 min rest).
  - Focus on pacing, strategy, and adapting to opponents.
- *Cooldown (15 min):* Stretching and foam rolling.

Saturday: Recovery and Mental Training
- *Active Recovery (30 min):* Light yoga or swimming.
- *Mental Training (30 min):* Visualization exercises, meditation, or mental rehearsal of techniques.

Sunday: Rest Day
- Focus on overall recovery, hydration, and nutrition.

Additional Considerations
- *Nutrition:* Prioritize a nutrient-dense diet with sufficient protein for muscle recovery, complex carbohydrates for energy, and healthy fats.
- *Supplementary Skills:* Consider cross-training in sports like wrestling, boxing, or Brazilian Jiu-Jitsu for additional skill enhancement.
- *Rest and Recovery:* Ensure adequate sleep and consider massage or physical therapy as needed.

Feel free to adapt this course to your specific needs, goals, or any particular skills you wish to enhance!

UGA KILLER CARDIO LEGS

1 x - Beginners / 3 x's – Intermediate / 5 x's Advanced

1. Run 10 Laps
2. Run Lines (Suicides)
3. Run in Place 1 Minute
4. 30 Mountain Climbers
5. 50 Squats
6. Walking Lunges
7. 50 Calf Raises
8. 50 Squats
9. 30 Side Lunges
10. 50 Calf Raises
11. 50 Crab Squats
12. 25 Kick Backs
13. 25 Doggie Straight Leg Raises

UGA FIGHTERS KILLER CARDIO

1 Minute – Beginners / 2 Minutes – Intermediate / 3 Minutes – Advanced

1. Cardio Machine
2. Pummeling
3. Bag Strikes
4. Greco Hands
5. Bag Strikes
6. Cardio Machine
7. Push-ups
8. Pummeling
9. Bag Strikes
10. Run in Place

11. Jumping Jacks
12. Bag Kicks
13. Cardio Machine
14. Push-ups
15. Greco Hands
16. Bag Strikes
17. Jumping Jacks
18. Shoulder Rolls

90 SECONDS of HITTING BAGS

Beginners 1 -2 Sets / Intermediate 2 – 4 / Sets Advanced 4 – 6 Sets

1. 90 Seconds of bags – Switch to a different bag after each round.
2. 10 Hits on bags or pads, then 10 jumping jacks for 90 seconds.
3. 10 Hits on bags or pads (Can use partner's hands) – 10 pushups 90 seconds.
4. 20 Hits / 30 crunches each bag.
5. 50 Strikes on each bag.

90 SECONDS of ABDOMINALS

1. Bicycles
2. Scissors
3. Leg Raises / Up – Down – Out - In
4. Knee Touch Crunches
5. Bruce Lee – Heal Touches
6. Model Pose Crunches

90 SECONDS of CARDIO

1. Bike - Slow Peddle / Fast Peddle
2. Cross Trainer – Slow Go / Fast Go
3. Treadmill – Walk / Run
4. Battle Ropes – 90 seconds

5. Run in Place – 90 seconds

THE 90 SECOND WORKOUT

Beginner 1-3 sets / Intermediate 4 -6 sets / Experienced 7 – 9 sets

1. 6 Laps
2. Jump Rope
3. Jumping Jacks
4. Squats
5. Shoulder Rolls Forward / Backwards
6. Pushups
7. Crunches
8. Mountain Climbers
9. Lunges
10. Plank

100 Rep Shoulder Workout

20 Repetitions per Exercise / 3 - 9 Sets

1. Press
2. Side Lateral
3. Arnold Press
4. Alternating Front Raise
5. Upright Rows

UGA - Burn Out – Work Out

Beginners: 3 Sets / 90 Second Rounds
Intermediate: 3 Sets / 2 Minute Rounds
Advanced: 3 Sets / 5 Minute Rounds

1. Squats
2. Head Punches

3. Bag Kicks
4. Medicine Ball Press
5. Push-Ups
6. Bent-Over Rows
7. Planks

Additional Exercises
Abdominal Exercises – Crunches, Leg Raises
Legs – Lunges or Leg Press
Curls – Barbell or Dumbbell Hammer
Triceps – Pushdowns or French Curls
Pull Downs

Speed Bag / Ride Bike / Cross Trainer / Treadmill

UGA - Killing It with Weights

Use Light to Moderate Weights
Practice Proper Form and Control over Weights or Machines
Stay Hydrated in-between Sets

Take 1 or More Exercises from Each Body Group or do 1 Whole Body Part and Perform 3 to 6 Sets of :
Repetitions: Beginners – Sets of 50 / Intermediate – Sets of 100 / Advanced - 150

Legs – Squats / Leg Extension / Hamstring Curls / Leg Press / Lunges / Calf Raises
Back – Pull Downs / Dead Lifts / Bent Over Rows / Seated Rows / Dumbbell Rows / Shrugs
Chest – Incline Press / Bench Press / DB Flyes / Push-Ups / DB Press / Cable Cross Overs
Shoulders – BB Press / Arnold Press / Side Lateral Raise / DB Front Raise / Up-Right Rows /
Triceps – Push-Downs / Dips / French Curls / Kick-Backs
Biceps – BB Curls / Reverse Curls / Hammer Curls
Abs – Leg Raises / Crunches / Scissors / Plank / Heel Touch / Model Pose / Penguins / Jack-Knives

UGA - Wake Up WorkOut

Do 3 sets upon waking up and using the restroom
Rest 30 seconds to 1 minute in between sets
After completion, drink a full class of water / protein drink, shower and enjoy your day.

1. 30 Jumping Jacks

2. 10 Pushups
3. 20 Crunches
4. 10 Pushups
5. 20 Calf Raises
6. 20 Squats
7. 10 High Knees
8. 20 Squats
9. 10 Pushups
10. 30 Jumping Jacks
11. 20 Squats
12. 20 Crunches
13. 1 Minute Plank

UGA - Daily Ten Work-Out

Do 3 or more sets with a 1-minute break in between sets

Morning Work-Out
Wake Up / Drink 1 Glass of Water / Use Restroom / Start Workout

1. 10 Jumping Jacks
2. 10 Burpees
3. 10 Crunches
4. 10 Front Lunges
5. 10 Side Lunges
6. 10 Push-Ups
7. 10 Dips
8. 10 Squats
9. 10 Calf Raises
10. 10 Knee Lifts
11. 10 Mountain Climbers
12. 1 Minute Plank

UGA - 20's 4 Life WorkOut

Level 1 – 3 Sets with 1 minute rest in between.
Level 2 – 6 Sets with 1 minute rest in between.
Level 3 – 9 Sets with 1 minute rest in between.

1. 20 Box Jumps
2. 20 Squats
3. 20 Lunges
4. 20 Close-Grip Push-Ups
5. 20 Leg Raises
6. 20 Cross-Shoulder Touches (High Plank Position)
7. 20 Sitting Twists (Russian Twists)
8. 20 Crunches
9. 20 Pull-Ups or Pull Downs

UGA - Calorie Blast Workout

60 seconds Each / 3 Times Around with 2 Minute Break

1. Jumping Jacks
2. Tricep Dips
3. Walking Lunges
4. Calf Raises
5. Mountain Climbers
6. Push Ups – On Knees
7. Plank
8. Squat Jumps
9. Crunches

UGA - Body WorkOut

1. 10 Burpees

2. 15 Pushups
3. 20 Crunches
4. 25 Squats
5. 30 Lunges
6. 35 Tricep Dips
7. 40 Mountain Climbers
8. 45 Sumo Squats
9. 50 Jumping Jacks
10. 60 Second Wall Sits

Repeat 3 times / 5 Minute Cool Down / Stretch

UGA Body Workout 2

Repeat workout 3 Times

1. 50 jumping Jacks
2. 10 Push-ups
3. 10 Russian Twists
4. 40 Sit Ups
5. 40 Lunges
6. 10 Squats
7. 30 Leg Crunches
8. 30 Jumping Jacks
9. 30 Superman
10. 10 Tricep Dips
11. 10 Side Lunges
12. 10 Push-ups
13. 20 KickBacks
14. 50 Bicycles
15. 50 Jumping Jacks

UGA Cardio-Challenge

Do 2 - 6 sets

1. 40 Jumping Jacks
2. 30 Second Jump Rope
3. 20 High Knees
4. 20 Butt Kickers
5. 30 Mountain Climbers
6. 5 Jump Squats
7. 5 Burpees
8. 30 Second Jump Rope
9. 30 - 60 Second Water Break
10. 25 Jumping Jacks
11. 20 Pivoting Upper cuts
12. 30 Second Run in Place
13. 5 Burpees
14. 35 Jumping Jacks
15. 40 Jump Rope
16. 5 Jump Squats
17. 30 High Knees

UGA - WEEKLY WORKOUT

Monday / Wednesday / Friday

1. 50 Squats
2. 50 Lunges
3. 50 Bent-Over Rows
4. 50 Deadlifts
5. 50 Shoulder Press
6. 50 Side Lateral Raises

7. 50 Incline Press
8. 50 DB Flyes
9. 50 Barbell Curls
10. 50 Hammer Curls

Tuesday / Thursday

1. 1 hour of Cardio - Non-Stop
2. 50 Calf Raises
3. 50 Superman
4. 50 Close Push-Ups
5. 50 Dips
6. 50 Forearm Exercises

Drink plenty of water, and take in high protein and amino acids. Eat a minimum of 3 to 6 modest meals daily. Drink 1 glass of water before each meal. Eat lean meat, fruits, and leafy green vegetables.

Avoid sugar drinks and food, milk, Juices, Starches.

UGA Spartan Training Routine

A 12-Week Program to Develop endurance, Strength, agility, and mental toughness.

Weekly Training Schedule
Train: 5 days a week (with 2 rest or active recovery days)

Day 1: Strength Training

Warm-Up: Our UGA Spartan training routine involves a mix of strength, endurance, and agility workouts, along with specific skills training to tackle obstacles. Here's a comprehensive 12-week training plan to get you ready:

Weeks 1-4: Foundation Building

Monday: Strength Training
- *Squats:* 3 sets of 10-12 reps
- *Push-ups:* 3 sets of 10-15 reps
- *Deadlifts:* 3 sets of 10 reps
- *Plank:* 3 sets of 30-60 seconds

Tuesday: Endurance Run
- 3-5 miles at a comfortable pace

Wednesday: Obstacle Skills
- Practice climbing (walls, ropes)
- Carrying weights (sandbags, buckets)
- Monkey bars or similar grip training

Thursday: Cross-Training
- Swimming, cycling, or rowing for 30-45 minutes

Friday: Strength Training
- *Lunges:* 3 sets of 10-12 reps per leg
- *Pull-ups:* 3 sets of 5-10 reps (or assisted)
- *Kettlebell swings:* 3 sets of 15 reps
- *Side plank:* 3 sets of 30 seconds per side

Saturday: Long Endurance Run
- 5-7 miles at a steady pace

Sunday: Rest and Recovery
- Light stretching or yoga

Weeks 5-8: Building Intensity

Monday: *High-Intensity Interval Training (HIIT)*
- 30 seconds of burpees, 30 seconds rest (repeat for 15-20 minutes)
- 400m sprint x 4 with rest in between

Tuesday: Strength & Obstacle Course
- Circuit training combining strength exercises with obstacle drills (e.g., jump over barriers, crawl under obstacles)

Wednesday: Endurance Run
- 4-6 miles with some hill work

Thursday: Cross-Training
- Engage in a different sport or activity that challenges your body (e.g., rock climbing, martial arts)

Friday: Strength Training
- *Barbell squats:* 4 sets of 8-10 reps
- *Box jumps:* 3 sets of 10 reps
- *Push-ups with a clap:* 3 sets of 8-10 reps
- *Core workout* (Russian twists, mountain climbers)

Saturday: Long Run with Obstacles
- 6-8 miles with some hills and obstacle practice

Sunday: Active Recovery
- Light jogging or walking, followed by stretching

Weeks 9-12: Race Simulation

Monday: Strength and Speed Work
- Combine heavy lifts with speed work (e.g., deadlifts followed by sprints)

Tuesday: Obstacle Course Race Simulation
- Create a mock race with various obstacles and run through it

Wednesday: Endurance Run
- 5-7 miles with tempo runs included

Thursday: Cross-Training
- Focus on mobility and flexibility (yoga or Pilates)

Friday: Strength Training
- Compound exercises focusing on functional strength (overhead press, farmer's carry)

Saturday: Long Distance with Speed Work
- 8-10 miles incorporating intervals (e.g., sprint for 1 minute every mile)

Sunday: Tapering and Recovery
Light activity, focus on rest and nutrition to prepare for race day

Additional Tips:

- **Nutrition:** Focus on a balanced diet rich in proteins, healthy fats, and carbs for energy.
- **Hydration:** Stay well-hydrated, especially during longer workouts.
- **Rest:** Listen to your body and allow for adequate recovery to prevent injury.
- **Mental Preparation:** Incorporate visualization techniques and positive affirmations as race day approaches.

Increasing Your Energy Levels

1. Get 6-8 Hours of sleep each night.
2. Drink plenty of water.
3. Drink Vegetable Juice.

4. Reduce Carbohydrate consumption.
5. Eat Chia Seeds.
6. Stay hydrated.
7. Get enough Vitamin B-12 / Take Multi-Vitamins with high vitamin B dosages.
8. Drink Herbal Tea.
9. Inhale or Diffuse peppermint oil.
10. Consume Adaptogenic Herbs – Ginseng, Sage, Guarana, Maca, Rosemary, Ashwagandha
11. Exercise Daily – Like joining the UGA adult program…
12. Avoid eating junk food.
13. Do Yoga
14. Eat Nuts.
15. Do not smoke.
16. Try essential Oils -
17. Drink Aloe Vera juice.
18. Snack on Cucumber and or Celery.
19. Limit alcohol.
20. Keep stress levels down. Relax, meditate, etc.

One of the main reasons for fatigue is "Overwork". Overwork can include professional, family, and social obligations. Try to streamline your list of "Must Do" activities. Set your priorities in terms of the most important tasks. Pare down those that are less important. Consider asking for extra help where needed, if necessary.

Exercise almost guarantees that you'll sleep more soundly. It also gives your cells more energy to burn and circulates oxygen. And exercising can lead to higher brain dopamine levels, which helps elevate mood. When walking, pick up the pace periodically to get extra health benefits and push your barriers to the next level.

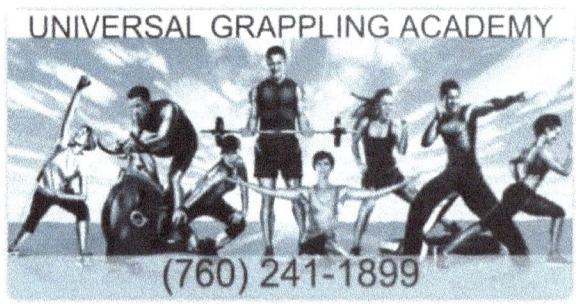

www.UniversalGrapplingAcademy.com

WEEKLY WORKOUT

MONDAY
100 jumping jacks
20 crunches
20 tricep dips
15 squats
20 lunges (ea leg)
70 Russian twists
20 standing calf rises
5 push-ups
30 seconds plank
10 lunge split jumps

TUESDAY
80 jumping jacks
50 vertical leg crunches
20 sit-ups
15 tricep dips
20 squats
10 side lunges (ea leg)
15 leg lifts (ea leg)
50 bicycles
15 wall push-ups
50 Russian twists

WEDNESDAY
90 jumping jacks
20 tricep dips
10 sit-ups
30 bird-dogs
30 seconds plank
30 squats
15 incline push-ups
40 crunches
10 oblique crunches (ea side)
20 standing calf rises

THURSDAY
100 jumping jacks
25 vertical leg crunches
30 crunches
20 squats
20 wall push-ups
50 Russian twists
15 second side plank (ea side)
10 lunge split jumps
5 jump squads
40 high knees

FRIDAY
60 jumping jacks
40 crunches
10 sit-ups
10 tricep dips
20 side lunges (ea side)
15 incline push-ups
10 oblique crunches (ea side)
30 butt kickers
5 jump squats
15 jack knife sit-ups

SATURDAY
50 jumping jacks
20 squats
100 Russian twists
5 kneeling push-ups
1 minute downward dog
15 jack knife sit-ups
10 lunges (ea leg)
10 side lunges (ea side)
20 bird-dogs
20 inner thigh lifts (ea leg)

SUNDAY
45 jumping jacks
15 squats
5 jump squats
50 Russian twists
30 seconds plank
10 standing calf rises
5 kneeling push-ups
30 seconds Superman
10 lunges (ea leg)
40 crunches

7 Day Workout

CrossFit Training

It's designed to improve strength, endurance, and overall fitness.
Warm-Up (10-15 minutes)

1. 5-10 minutes of light cardio (jogging, rowing, or jumping rope)
2. Stretches:
  - *Arm circles* (30 seconds)
  - *Leg swings* (30 seconds each leg)
  - *Hip circles* (30 seconds each direction)
  - *Spidermans* (10 reps each side)

Strength Training (20-30 minutes)
Choose one of the following lifts:
- *Back Squat:* 5 sets of 5 reps
- *Deadlift:* 5 sets of 5 reps
- *Shoulder Press:* 5 sets of 5 reps

Workout of the Day (WOD) (15-20 minutes)
AMRAP (As Many Rounds As Possible) in 15 minutes:
- 5 Pull-ups
- 10 Push-ups
- 15 Weightless Squats
- Short run

Cool Down (5-10 minutes)
- Stretch major muscle groups (hold each stretch for about 30 seconds)
- Focus on areas that feel tight or sore

Weightless Routine

A weightless training routine can focus on bodyweight exercises, which effectively build strength, flexibility, and endurance without the need for equipment.

Warm-Up (5-10 minutes)

1. *Jumping Jacks* - 2 minutes
2. *Arm Circles* - 1 minute (30 seconds forward, 30 seconds backward)
3. *Leg Swings* - 1 minute (30 seconds each leg)
4. *Stretching* - 2-3 minutes (e.g., walking lunges, high knees)

Full-Body Workout (30-40 minutes)
Perform 2-3 sets of each exercise, resting 30-60 seconds between sets.

1. *Push-Ups* - 10-15 reps
2. *Squats* - 15-20 reps
3. *Plank* - Hold for 30-60 seconds
4. *Lunges* - 10-15 reps per leg
5. *Burpees* - 8-12 reps
6. *Mountain Climbers* - 30 seconds
7. *Glute Bridges* - 15-20 reps
8. *Tricep Dips* (using a chair or bench) - 10-15 reps

Core Workout (10-15 minutes)
1. *Bicycle Crunches* - 15-20 reps
2. *Leg Raises* - 10-15 reps
3. *Side Plank* - Hold for 20-30 seconds on each side
4. *Russian Twists* - 15-20 reps

Cool Down (5-10 minutes)
1. Stretching - Focus on major muscle groups (hamstrings, quadriceps, shoulders, etc.)
2. Deep Breathing Exercises - 3-5 minutes to relax your body and mind.

Speed & Agility WorkOut
A speed and agility workout focuses on improving your quickness, coordination, and overall athletic performance.

Warm-Up (5-10 minutes)
1. Stretching - Focus on legs, hips, and shoulders (e.g., leg swings, arm circles).
2. High Knees - 1 minute
3. Butt Kickers - 1 minute
4. Side Shuffles - 1 minute

Speed Drills (20-25 minutes)
1. Sprints - 5-10 x 100 feet (focus on explosive starts; walk back to recover between sprints).
2. A-Skip - 3 sets of 65 feet (focus on knee drive and proper form).
3. B-Skip - 3 sets of 65 feet (extend leg and swing it back down).
4. Bounding - 3 sets of 65 feet (long strides, focusing on distance).
5. Acceleration Drills - 5 x 10-100 feet (start from a standing position and sprint).

Agility Drills (20-25 minutes)
1. Ladder Drills (if you have an agility ladder):
   - *In-and-Outs* - 2 sets of 30 seconds
   - *Lateral Shuffles* - 2 sets of 30 seconds
   - *Ali Shuffle* - 2 sets of 30 seconds

2. Cone Drills:
   - *T-Drill:* Set up 4 cones in a T-shape. Sprint to the middle cone, shuffle to each side, then backpedal to the start. Repeat 3-5 times.
   - *Box Drill:* Place cones in a square. Sprint to each cone and back to the center. Repeat for 3-5 minutes.

3. Zig-Zag Runs - Set up cones in a zig-zag pattern and sprint through them. Repeat 3-5 times.

Cool Down (5-10 minutes)
1. Static Stretching - Focus on legs, hips, and lower back.
2. Deep Breathing Exercises - 3-5 minutes to help lower your heart rate.

Tips:
- Focus on form and technique during drills to maximize benefits.
- Incorporate this workout 2-3 times per week for optimal improvement.
- Make sure to stay hydrated and listen to your body to avoid injury.

Enjoy your training!

UGA DRILLS

Takedowns, Spin Drills, Reversals, Take Down against Cage/Wall, Stand ups against Cage/Walls, Partner on your back - Stand Ups, Full Mount Escapes, Side Mount Escapes, Back Mount Escapes, Guard Escapes, Wheel Barrels, Shoot/Sprawl, Spider Mans,

KIDS Warm-Ups

1. Begin with Jogging
2. Walk/Run Backwards
3. Cross Overs
4. Step and Slide
5. Bear Crawls
6. Military Crawls
7. Worm Drills/Shrimps
8. Mountain Climbers
9. Frog Leaps
10. Front Rolls / Back Rolls
11. Lunge Walks
12. Jumping Jacks, Sprawls, and Push-Ups
13. Partner Drills: Single Leg, Double Leg, Tie Up Take downs, Duck-Under(s, Side Mount, Full Mount, Front Chokes, Back Chokes, Triangle Choke, Arm Bars from Full - Side Mounts, Bottom and North/South Positions.

UGA Kids in Shape

A 30 Minute Cardio and Conditioning Work-Out for Children

30 / 20 / 10

1. Runs or other Cardio Exercise (Laps, Suicides, etc.)
2. Jumping Jacks
3. Sumo - Squats
4. Lunges

5. Mountain Climbers
6. Push-Ups
7. Crunches
8. Strikes (Punches, Kicks, Knees, and Elbows)

Develop Strength, Speed, Agility, Flexibility, and Endurance

UGA Adults in Shape

A 45-Minute Cardio and Conditioning Work-Out for Adults

100 / 80 / 40 / 20 / 10

1. Runs, Suicides, or other Cardio Exercises
2. Jumping Jacks
3. Crunches
4. Squats
5. Leg Lifts
6. 1 Minute Plank

Develop Strength, Speed, Agility, Flexibility, and Endurance

Functional Training Routine for Combat Sports

Creating a functional training routine for combat sports athletes involves focusing on strength, agility, endurance, and flexibility. This routine is designed to enhance overall athletic performance, focusing on the essential attributes for combat sports.

Warm-Up (10-15 Minutes):
1. Dynamic Stretching (5-7 minutes)
 - Arm circles
 - Leg swings
 - Torso twists

2. Agility Drills (5-8 minutes)
 - Ladder drills
 - Cone sprints (forward, lateral, backward)

Strength Training (30-40 Minutes):
1. Compound Movements (3 sets of 8-12 reps each)

- Squats (barbell or bodyweight)
- Deadlifts (traditional or sumo)
- Bench Press or Push-Ups
- Pull-Ups or Bent-over Rows

2. Functional Strength (3 sets of 10-15 reps each)
- Kettlebell swings
- Medicine ball slams
- Turkish get-ups

Conditioning (20-30 Minutes):
1. High-Intensity Interval Training (HIIT)
- 30 seconds of work followed by 30 seconds of rest, repeat for 15-20 minutes:
  - Burpees
  - Shadow boxing with intensity
  - Jump rope
  - Mountain climbers

2. Sport-Specific Drills (10 minutes)
- Footwork drills specific to the combat sport (e.g., boxing, MMA)
- Sparring or partner drills focusing on technique and timing

Core Training (15 Minutes):
1. Plank Variations (3 sets of 30-60 seconds each)
- Standard plank
- Side planks (both sides)
- Plank with shoulder taps

2. Rotational Exercises (3 sets of 10-15 reps each)
- Russian twists
- Medicine ball rotational throws

Cool Down (10-15 Minutes):
1. Stretching (hold each stretch for 20-30 seconds)
- Hamstring stretch
- Quadriceps stretch
- Shoulder and triceps stretch
- Hip flexor stretch

2. Breathing Exercises
- Deep breathing to promote relaxation and recovery.

Notes:
- Adjust the intensity and volume based on the athlete's training phase.
- Ensure proper hydration and nutrition to support training demands.
- Incorporate rest days and recovery sessions to prevent injuries.

50 Rep Full Body Weightless Workout

3 sets - Beginners / 6 sets - Intermediate / 9 sets Advanced

1. Warm-Up: Jog, jump rope, or run in place
2. 50 walking lunges
3. 50 squats
4. 50 calf raises
5. 50 shoulder press
6. 50 side lateral raises
7. 50 push-ups
8. 50 dips
9. 50 bent-over rows
10. 50 deadlifts or super-mans
11. 50 curls
12. 50 hammer curls
13. 50 alternating wrist curls
14. 50 crunches

Power Lifting for Life

4 - 8 sets / 6 - 8 heavy reps / 3 days per week

Alternate Option - Do 1 exercise each day for 5 days, executing 1 50-rep warm-up set, 6 - 8 sets of 6-8 reps with heavy weight.

1. Warm up for each exercise with a 50-rep set
2. Squats
3. Dead-Lifts
4. Shoulder Press
5. Dumbbell Press or Flies
6. Curls

Hotel Workout Routine

On the Road Workout

Staying active while traveling can be challenging, but with a hotel workout routine, you can maintain your fitness. Here's a simple yet effective routine you can do while on the road. You can use the hotel gymnasiums as well.

Warm-Up (5-10 minutes)
- *Jumping jacks:* 2 minutes
- *Arm circles:* 1 minute (30 seconds forward, 30 seconds backward)
- *Leg swings:* 1 minute (30 seconds each leg)

Circuit (Repeat 2-3 times)
1. *Bodyweight Squats:* 15-20 reps
2. *Push-Ups:* 10-15 reps (modify by doing them on your knees if needed)
3. *Plank:* Hold for 30 seconds to 1 minute
4. *Lunges:* 10 reps per leg
5. *Tricep Dips:* 10-15 reps (use a sturdy chair or bed)
6. *Mountain Climbers:* 30 seconds

Cool Down (5-10 minutes)
- *Stretching:* Focus on major muscle groups (hold each stretch for 15-30 seconds)
- *Deep breathing exercises* to relax

Extra Tips:
- Use hotel furniture for added resistance (e.g., chairs for dips).
- If available, incorporate resistance bands or dumbbells into the routine.
- Stay hydrated and listen to your body; adjust the reps and sets based on your fitness level.

This workout can be completed in about 30-45 minutes, making it easy to fit into your travel schedule!

What you think you're paying for when taking a UGA-MMA Class

* Being taught to exercise, grapple and strike.

THE MANY THINGS YOU REALLY GETTING WHEN JOINING A UGA-MMA CLASS

* A life coach.
* A Combat Sports Coach to teach you how to exercise, grapple and strike.
* Mentor.
* A psychologist/Psychiatrist.
* An Inspirer.
* A Supporter.
* A Friend.
* A Problem Solver.
* A Stress Reliever.
* Someone to encourage your self belief.
* A Nutritionist and Personal Trainer.
* Strength, Flexibility, Discipline and Weight Management.
* Personal Achievements and Victories.
* Someone to encourage your children and yourself to have Respect, Patience, Humility, Courage, Loyalty, Perseverance, Empathy, Listening Skills, and Self Control.
* Someone to Encourage You and your Children to Train Hard & Finish Strong.
* Lessons on how Hard Work Pays Off and How to Enjoy Life.
* Lessons on How to be Accountable for Your Actions.
* Learning Successful Goal Setting and Reaching Them.
* Someone who helps you build Mental, Physical and Emotional Strength.
* Team Building Skills.
* Someone who'll Teach You to Stand Up for Yourself against Bullies.
* Someone who'll Pick You Up when You're Down.
* Martial Arts Knowledge, Wisdom, Opportunities and More.
* An Instructor who's spent his life training to assist you and put his heart/soul in to your training and goals.

So if you think you're paying too much for UGA-MMA classes, Think Again!
No other professional offers everything that you'll get here for this low cost.

Final words from the Coach

Thank you, and Congratulations to all the readers of the UGA Athletes' Training Guide! Your commitment to enhancing your knowledge and skills is commendable, and I hope you've absorbed valuable insights or refreshed essential elements of your training. Regardless of where you are in your journey, you are now and forever a part of the UGA family—an integral part of our mental, physical, and educational lineage. It is my sincere hope that I have contributed positively to your health, fitness, training, confidence, or knowledge. If you find that my efforts have made a difference, please share your experiences with me and, even more importantly, let others know. Together, we can continue to uplift and inspire our combat sports community in the UGA way.

Book 1 of our MMA & Fitness Series

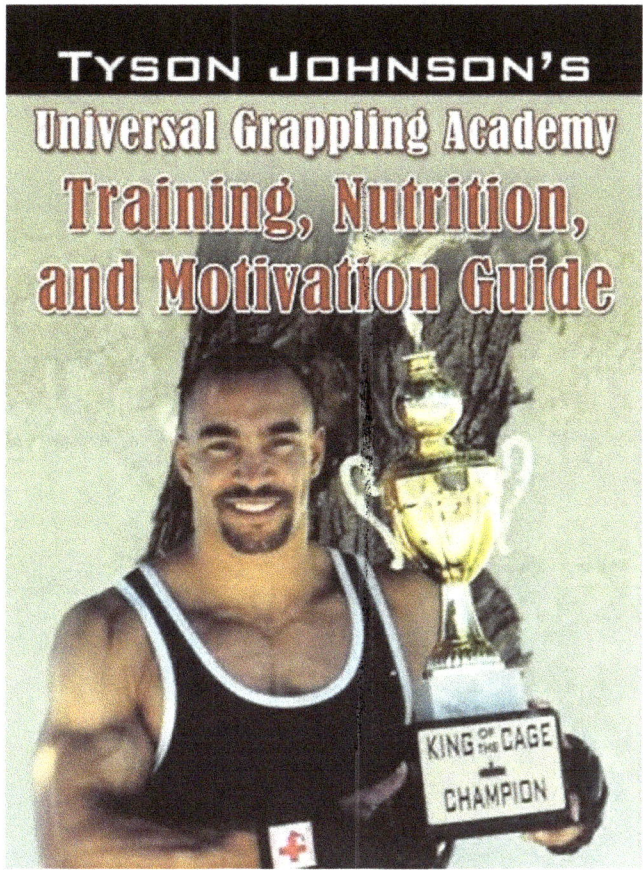

Available at Amazon.com

Book 2 of our MMA & Fitness Series

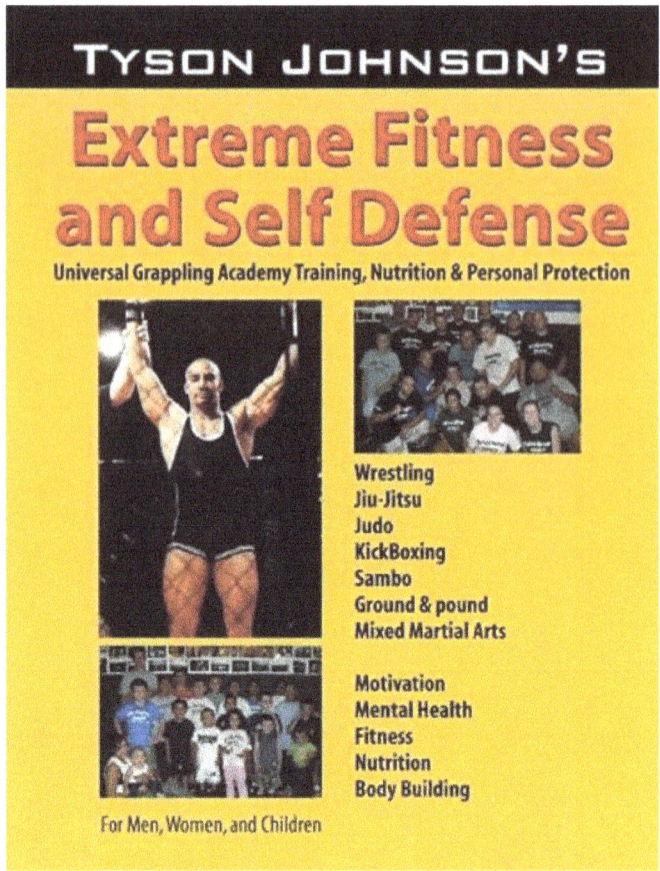

Available at Amazon.com

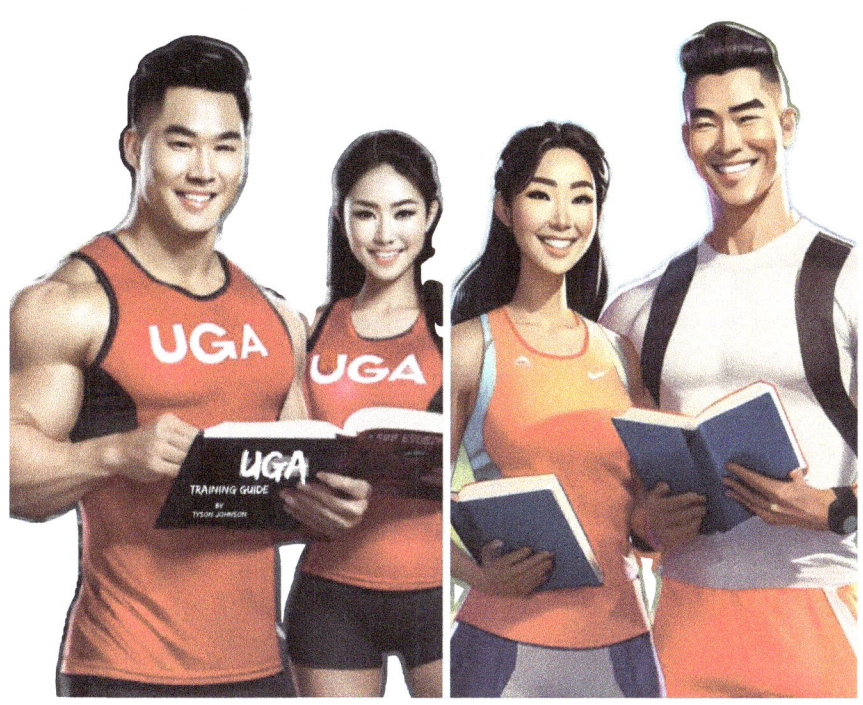

What Many People Are Saying

1. Transformative Experience!
"The Universal Grappling Academy is a game-changer! Tyson Johnson's books on training and nutrition have completely transformed my approach to mixed martial arts. His insights are not just for seasoned fighters; they're accessible for beginners too. The Academy's environment is supportive, and the coach genuinely cares about everyone's growth. Highly recommend for anyone looking to elevate their skills!"

2. Empowering for All Ages!
"Tyson Johnson's books are a fantastic resource for families! My kids and I have been training at the Universal Grappling Academy, and we all benefit from the self-defense techniques and nutritional advice. The lessons are engaging and tailored for all ages, making it easy for us to learn together. This is more than just martial arts; it's a journey of empowerment!"

3. Comprehensive and Practical!
"As a long-time practitioner of combat sports, I've read many training books, but Tyson Johnson's works stand out for their practicality and depth. The Universal Grappling Academy embodies the principles he teaches, offering hands-on experience that complements the reading. The nutrition tips have helped me optimize my performance. If you're serious about MMA, this is essential reading!"

4. Inspiring and Motivating!
"Walking into the Universal Grappling Academy felt like home! Tyson Johnson's motivational writing shines through in his books, which encourage a healthy lifestyle and commitment to training. His focus on mental strength alongside physical conditioning has inspired me to push my limits. The community here is incredible — I've made lifelong friends while learning invaluable skills!"

5. A Holistic Approach to Fitness!
"Tyson Johnson's books are a treasure trove of knowledge! The way he integrates training, nutrition, and self-defense is refreshing and effective. At the Universal Grappling Academy, I've learned not just how to fight, but how to live a healthier life. The classes cater to everyone, making it a welcoming space for men, women, and kids alike. Highly recommend for anyone looking to enhance their fitness journey!"

6. Exceptional Coaching and Resources!
"The Universal Grappling Academy sets the standard for martial arts training! Tyson Johnson's books are the perfect companion to the classes offered here, providing in-depth knowledge on combat sports and effective nutrition. The coach is incredibly skilled and attentive, ensuring that everyone improves at their own pace. Whether you're a novice or an expert, there's something here for everyone!"

7. A Must for Aspiring Fighters!
"If you're serious about mixed martial arts, you need to check out the Universal Grappling Academy! Tyson Johnson's books are filled with actionable insights that I've applied in my training. The blend of technique, nutrition, and self-defense makes for a comprehensive learning experience. Plus, the atmosphere is electric! I've never felt more motivated to become the best version of myself."

Hey Tyson I see you still doing your thing I just want to thank you for taking my son Anthony Whitfield (scooter) under your wing. Years of your guidance, discipline and teaching has really brung so much positive in my son life. One of the best choices ever made. He's really good at this MMA I will always be his biggest fan, best friend and mother. Due to circumstances I have not been able to attend his matches but I help promote and gather family and friends there for my sons support team. I'm really proud of my kiddo and I just wanted to say thank you   **January 11, 2025**

On this day
12 years ago

Jamal Pogues is with **Tyson Johnson** and **Nelson Alvarado**.
Dec 4, 2012

I have good team and a coach behind me helping me get ready for my fight. I had some days when I wanted to quit but I knew eventually I would have regretted on my decision and wasted my time and my teammates. In these last 12 days for my fight I wanna say thank you for turning me into a better fighter I was 2 months ago.

Jennifer Morales ▸ **Tyson Johnson**
Aug 30, 2012

Thank youuu you r TOTALLY   the best coach ever !!!!!!!!!!!!<3333333

This fire that's in me was inspired by @universal_grappling_academy for making me one of their own & tyson supporting me each day to be a fighter & get my weight & endurance in check, only way from here is up !!

Emit Gomez Monday April 11, 2022

Your awesome coach you and taught my boys How to defend themselves not be bullies at a young age me and Janette will always be grateful for that

super excited today coach, ill try to get some sleep in before training but im coming ready, just wanted to say thank you, you really made me want to be my best self with all the positive reinforcement you've been giving me & support, see you tonight ! 🥊🥋

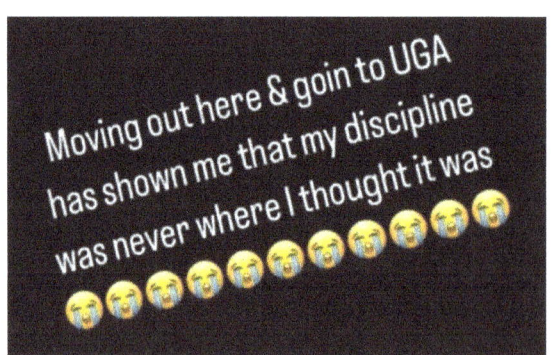

I love you, I respect you, and I'm grateful to have you as a coach, role model, and a mentor. Thank you for everything you've done for me I appreciate you.

Rob Longoria
Uga Mma Tyson Johnson best in the hd treat you like family it's an amazing program

13h   Like   Reply

Kathy Elden Nielsen
Uga Mma is the absolute best ever! Tyson Johnson is the man.

12h   Like   Reply

Joseph Rogers
Uga Mma best kids program in this desert hands down

> Hey coach I just wanted to send you some words because I don't tell you enough. Where I am in life is because of meeting you and learning that although life is hard it isn't going anywhere. Facing your battles and demons is what UGA taught me!!
> Your more of a role model to me mari and the kids then you could imagine coach.
>
> I just want to say thank you coach and that we love you!!! 😊

Caitlin Sanchez

This young man is slaying life! Was proud of his time spent at UGA and proud of him now! Thanks Tyson for being a great influence in his life ❤️

Mandee Martin

We love you so much coach! You are our family. I'm so glad my boys have you in their lives, you are an amazing example of what a man is and the greatest mentor. Merry Christmas coach and Happy New Year!!!

Just now   Love   Reply   1

Edward Bruns

Brother, you are the inspiration that drove me to coach when the opportunity arose, you have always busted your ass and hustled, and i hope to be half the Coach you have been, and are today. Thank you.

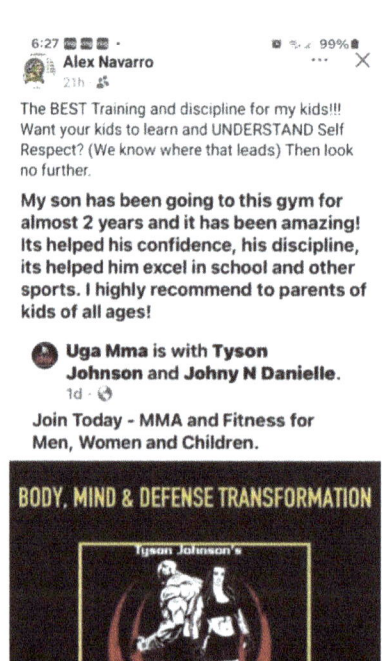

Carl Williams
Tyson Johnson UGA
Owner, fighter, coach who has trained fighters and future fighters, Is doing a fantastic job with young girs, boys and adults. I am so impressed with Tyson developing these girls. He as them daily training with the boys. He is getting great results..

May 2021

Life comes full circle. Today we signed the boys up at the same place I trained at years ago. Thank you Coach Tyson Johnson. The boys are very excited to get started and learn. It was also awesome catching up with my old Coach. #UGA

Sunday May 2, 2021

Started at 270 now Iam down to 253 thanks coach Tyson Johnson for setting the game plan and all the tips knowledge you been giving me and thanks Ashley Mora for helping me stick to it and always keeping me motivated and finding new healthy but bomb ass food to keep making none of this would of been possible if it wasent for you guys

---

Paola Cardoz Taylor
Love this ❤️
UGA = Family

I couldn't be more grateful for having these wonderful people in our lives. Uga Mma Valentines Practice lol

Time to get back on this grind Tyson Johnson thank you for always lifting my head up when it's down and never bullshitting me and telling me how it is....you Remind so much of my pops and that's why I love and respect you so much as a person.... now enough with the mushy shii I'll see you tonight coach thanks for always being their for me best thing I ever done was sign up for Uga Mma.... come join the squad if you ready for life changing experiences I promise you won't regret it

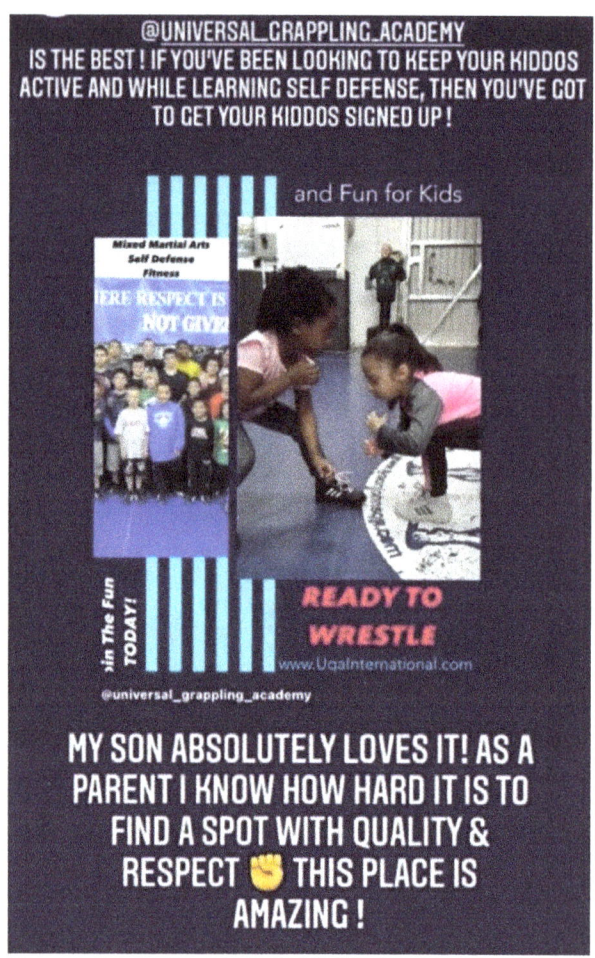

Will Navarro

This place you've created Mr. Johnson is home to a lot of people. You are a blessing to families and I am honored to call you friend. 👊

Kent Galloway

We love 💕 u Tyson Johnson. U r a fantastic person and a great example of what a REAL MAN should b. Caring, compassionate, and a moral example of a consummate Champion. And my own grasshopper. U make me proud and also proud to b in ur life.

6h Love Reply

Robin Galloway

💕Thank you for taking the time with us.. you are absolutely awesome 💕

.Thank you brother. They always come and tell me you did ask for me. They both enjoy going there and socializing with beautiful people. My daughter feel comfortable and she is seen how Jacob is improving not just physical but also mentally. I do really appreciate you for that and the kind of love you have for everyone there!! God bless you Tyson as He has done it until now. I love and respect you brother!💯

Christine Castro
Uga Mma hands down! You won't be disappointed. Very family oriented, coach is beyond amazing and the kids gain knowledge, strength, and encouragement to be confident in protecting themselves.

😂 i was not expecting that haha, its kinda unbelievable the amount of progress ive made in such a short time with a good coach, i seriously cannot thank you enough for my new skillsets & motivation you gave me tyson, i really do appreciate everything you've put into me (no homo) lmao, my only regret is not looking for a better gym the first time CK dicked me, now i got everyone tryinf to learn what you taught me & i feel like i found a gold mine at uga, you're the best tyson seriously 💚 **A.S. (Hercules) May 3, 2022**

I appreciate everything you do for the team at UGA! I couldnt have found a better place for my son

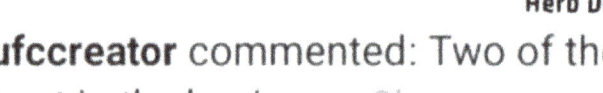

ufccreator commented: Two of the best in the business. 9h   July 2021

Herb Dean & Tyson Johnson

ABOUT THE AUTHOR

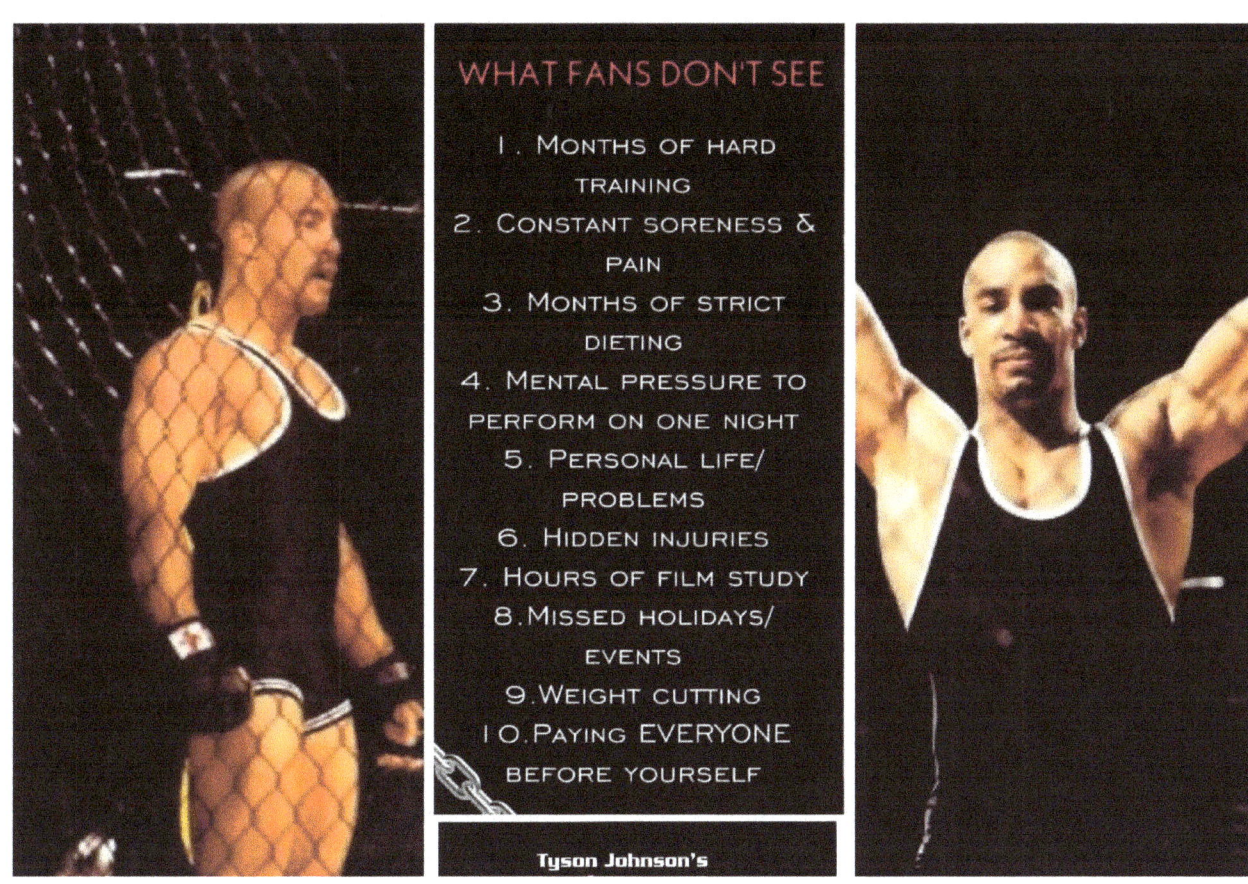

Tyson Johnson - Wrestling Champion, Bodybuilding Champion, Pit-Fighter, ToughMan Champion, Grappling Champion, Mixed Martial Arts Champion, 2008 USA Martial Arts Hall of Fame Inductee, 2013 USA Martial Arts Hall of Fame - Hall of Heroes Inductee, 2020 Lifetime Achievement Award. Ring/Cage Announcer, Author, Actor/Model. Trainer of Champions! Trainer of Multiple MMA Instructors, Certified Training and Nutritionist, Certified Peer Counselor, over 30 years in the Combat Sports Business.

BOOK DESCRIPTION

Unlock your potential and elevate your performance with "The UGA Athlete's Training Guide," a comprehensive resource crafted by expert coach Tyson Johnson. Designed for both new and seasoned athletes engaged in combat sports, this guide transcends the boundaries of the ring, offering invaluable insights applicable to any sport and personal endeavor.

Within these pages, you will discover the core principles of training, nutrition, and mental conditioning that define a champion's mindset. Tyson Johnson shares his wealth of experience and strategic wisdom, guiding you through tailored workouts, effective recovery techniques, and the mental fortitude required to overcome challenges in the Universal Grappling Academy, in competition, and in life.

Whether you're seeking to refine your skills in the octagon, improve your overall athleticism, or cultivate resilience and discipline in your daily routine, "The UGA Athlete's Training Guide" is your essential companion. Embrace the journey to greatness, and learn how the principles of the Universal Grappling Academy and combat sports can empower you to achieve success in all aspects of life. Transform your approach to training and develop the champion within!

www.ingramcontent.com/pod-product-compliance
Lightning Source LLC
Chambersburg PA
CBHW080947050426
42337CB00055B/4585